The Gourmet's Companion™
French
Menu Guide
&
Translator

Other Titles by Bernard Rivkin

The Gourmet's Companion: German Menu Guide & Translator
The Gourmet's Companion: Italian Menu Guide & Translator
The Gourmet's Companion: Spanish Menu Guide & Translator

The Author wishes to express appreciation to the French government tourist office for their cooperation and assistance, and the supply of some of the information used in the preparation of this book.

The Gourmet's Companion™
French
Menu Guide
&
Translator

Bernard Rivkin

John Wiley & Sons, Inc.

New York • Chichester • Brisbane • Toronto • Singapore

Copyright © 1991 by Bernard Rivkin of Bellaire Publishing
Published by John Wiley & Sons, Inc.
All rights reserved. Published simultaneously in Canada.

Library of Congress Cataloging-in-Publication Data

Rivkin, Bernard.
    The gourmet's companion: French menu guide and
      translator / Bernard Rivkin.
      p. cm.
    Includes bibliographical references.
    ISBN 0-471-52518-9
    1. Food—Dictionaries. 2. Cookery, French—Dictionaries.
3. Cookery—France. I. Title.
TX349.R49   1991
641.5944'03—dc20   90-38834

Printed in the United States of America
91 92 10 9 8 7 6 5 4 3 2 1

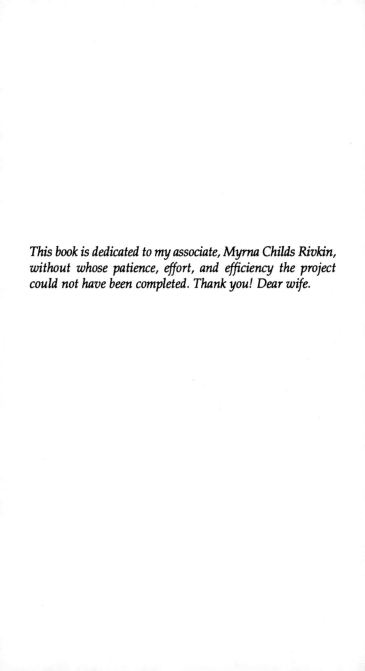

This book is dedicated to my associate, Myrna Childs Rivkin, without whose patience, effort, and efficiency the project could not have been completed. Thank you! Dear wife.

Contents

Food and Wine in France:
An Overview

General Notes

Dining pleasures in France can achieve unequaled heights. French cooking is made up of many different culinary styles which can be broadly described using the following categories:

- *Grande, Classic,* or *Haute cuisine,* which is rich, expensively and elaborately prepared, ornate, and generally better to look at than eat.

- *Nouvelle cuisine* became popular about 20 years ago as a result of popular demand for lighter food, in line with the concern for fitness. Preparation is simple, using seasonal and fresh ingredients. Cooking times are shortened, retaining the nutrients, natural flavors, and appearance. Lightness requires the very limited use of butter, cream, flour, fat, and alcohol.

- *Regional* or *Rustic* cooking includes old traditions. Since every 100 miles in France becomes a different region, with its own cooking style and special ingredients, regional food can be very unique and interesting. It should be experienced whenever possible.

- *Bistro* or *Cuisine Bourgeoise,* served in Paris and the bigger cities, is the type of food eaten every day and consists of long simmered dishes, most often found in little restaurants and bistros.

Manners and customs in France have some small differences. Dinner is eaten later and in a more leisurely manner. Dress is more formal for both men and women with ties and jackets for men and dressy attire for women.

The French usually have three meals a day: breakfast, lunch and dinner.

Breakfast is eaten between 6:30 and 9:00 a.m. It generally consists of black coffee and hot milk. Sometimes tea is taken, accompanied by bread, toast or croissants with butter and sometimes jam.

Lunch is generally the most important of the three meals. It is eaten between 12:30 p.m. or 1:00 p.m. and 3:00 p.m. Sometimes it is preceded by an aperitif. Lunch usually consists of an hors d'oeuvre, an entree of meat with a vegetable or some other side dish, some cheese, and dessert. The entire meal is accompanied by wine, beer, or mineral water. Lunch ends with coffee and, sometimes, a liqueur.

Dinner is more or less determined by working hours, but it often plays a part in the natural progression of the evening. It usually begins around 8:30 p.m. but can be eaten as late as 11:30 p.m., or even 1:00 a.m. The French refer to the very late dinner as *le souper*.

It should be noted that the French do not drink hot chocolate, coffee or coffee with milk with meals. Coffee comes afterwards and is considered to facilitate digestion. It is served quite strong, like Italian espresso. Salted foods are very rarely served along with sweet ones. Pickles and mayonnaise are never sweet, peanut butter does not exist, and ketchup is never used, except in such instances as with eggs and bacon, hamburgers, or steak tartare. These dishes are not considered to be part of French cooking, but are available in specialized restaurants such as *brasseries*, *drugstores*, or other fast-food establishments.

The Art of Good Eating in France

In France there are two distinct styles of eating. One is, of course, **gastronomy** which is widely known and deservedly famous. It is honored as an art and practiced as a cult, with its own rituals, rules, and taboos. But, it is only rarely practiced in daily life, partly because of the time which must be devoted to it, and mostly because of its rather high cost. A true gastronomic meal can cost between 500 to 1,000 FF, or even more, depending on the wines chosen to accompany it. Certain wines can cost 500 FF a bottle, or even more.

The other style is **family style cooking,** which is often just as delicious as its more celebrated counterpart, and can be very simple or very elegant. As its name indicates, it is the result of a carefully maintained family tradition. It is the style of cooking experienced daily by the majority of Frenchmen, and is heartily appreciated. Because it is the most common style of French cooking, it is the style most visitors to France will experience first. That is why it is emphasized here.

Tradition oriented chefs are members of **Les Cuisiniers et Hôteliers de Métier.** Just look for their plaques.

A note on tipping: Many menu prices include a service charge, others add 12, 15, or 18% to the bill. This is known as *service compris.* If no service has been added, 15% for more or less the caliber of service and price range of the meal should be left. If the wine steward and/or headwaiter have been particularly good, their service should be recognized with 10- to 20-franc tips.

The Menu

Almost all restaurants offer two types of meals: *à la carte* and *le menu.*

- Meals a la carte offer an extensive choice for each course, but this becomes more expensive, unless daily specials (dishes which are specially recommended and thus a bargain), are among the choices.

- The menu is a meal at a fixed price. Its dishes have been chosen from among those on the a la carte list. It usually consists of an appetizer, an entree (meat or fish), a vegetable, cheese, and/or a dessert. Within each course some choice is offered, allowing you some latitude in putting together a meal according to your own tastes from among the proposed dishes. The dinner also has a choice among two or three such menus for which the fixed prices vary according to the number of courses. The same meal chosen from the a la carte list can often cost as much as 30-40% more. Coffee is never included in the fixed price menu. It should also be noted that often in the countryside a **tourist** menu is offered. This means that wine and the tip are included in the fixed price.

What to Choose: Entrees

One of the dishes most often found on a fixed-price menu or on an a la carte listing in all typical restaurants is the inevitable steak with french fries, in all its variations: *tournedos* (small steaks ringed with bacon), *chateaubriand*, and *entrecôte* (rib steak). These are grilled or served with a sauce: *béarnaise* (a delicate sauce with an egg base), *bordelaise* (made with Bordeaux wine), *bercy* (made with red wine), or *marchand de vin* (the steak juices reduced with butter, chopped shallots and red wine). The French, however, prefer a host of other classic dishes such as:

- *Hachis parmentier* (meat and potato hash), *raie au beurre noir* (skate fish in brown butter), *daube de boeuf* (beef stew), *chou farci* (stuffed cabbage);

- *gigot de pré-salé* or leg of lamb, roasted or broiled, traditionally served along with *flageolets*, a type of kidney bean, or mashed potatoes, or *pommes dauphines* (deep fried mashed potato puffs), *gratin dauphinois* (scalloped potatoes made with truffles and cream);

- lamb chops served with green beans, or grilled with herbs and accompanied by tomatoes in the Provençal style (sautéed with garlic and herbs), or by *ratatouille niçoise*, a sort of stew of zucchini, tomatoes, and eggplant, all braised with garlic in olive oil;

- brochettes, in many combinations of cubes of meat or seafood on skewers, alternating with mushrooms, onions or tomatoes, which are grilled and served on rice;

- variety meats (offal), such as *andouillette* (a kind of chitterling sausage), grilled pigs' or calves' feet, *maître d'hôtel* calves' liver with lemon and butter, kidneys in Madeira sauce or with mustard, sweetbreads with bacon and peas, tripe, and blood sausage with applesauce;

- chicken, roasted and served garnished with watercress and sautéed potatoes, or in a sauce such as *coq au vin* (with red wine), or with rice in a white wine sauce, or hunter style (with mushrooms);

- rabbit, stewed with red wine, or with mustard and cream, or hunter style;

- the very popular *pot-au-feu*, beef boiled with vegetables and served with course salt, also known as *petite marmite*;

- mutton stew with potatoes and tomatoes, known as *navarin aux pommes* or *haricot de mouton* when it is made with kidney beans;

- slab-bacon served with lentils or cabbage; *daube*, beef simmered with red wine and carrots; *blanquette*, a veal stew with mushrooms in a white wine cream sauce.

All of these savory dishes should be tasted to get a good idea of what French family cooking is like.

Cheeses

France produces at least 347 different cheeses. Some of the better known are *Camembert*, *Brie*, *Roquefort* (to be eaten mixed with fresh butter), *Reblochon*, and blue cheeses from Auvergne and Bresse. Visitors to France should try to taste some of the lesser-known but equally delicious cheeses they may come across in their travels; *Banon* from Provence, *Chaource* from Burgundy, *Tomme* from Savoie, *Munster* from Alsace (sometimes spiced with cumin), *Fourme* from Ambert or Forez, *Picodon* from the Ardèche, and so many others—not to mention all the types of goat cheese with their picturesque names: *trouser buttons*, *Chabichou*, *Crottin* from Chavignol, *Rigotte* from Condrieux, *Pelardon*, *donkey-pepper*, and so on.

Desserts

Historically, and most particularly from the middle ages, France has been renowned for its creative genius in both foods and desserts. The French royal court introduced most of the more popular desserts which have filtered down to popular and continued use.

Light desserts include soufflé made with Grand Marnier, meringue with toasted almonds, *oeufs à la neige* (meringues floating on a custard lake), chocolate mousse, and pears *bourdaloue* (caramelized pears resting on a bed of vanilla cream).

Pastries include *mille-feuilles* (alternating layers of flaky pastry and custard cream), *puits d'amour* (caramel cream in a fine pastry crust); *éclairs*, *religieuses* (little balls of puff pastry, filled with cream), *Paris-Brest* (a large puff pastry with hazelnut cream), and *ganache* (a chocolate cream biscuit).

Tarts include strawberry, raspberry, blueberry, and so on; *tarte Tatin* (caramelized upside down apple tart).

Wine

Most restaurants have at least one *sommelier*, or wine steward, who will gladly give advice without trying to push expensive wines. The sommelier matches the wine to your taste preferences and the food ordered. France produces thousands of unique wines, some which never leave the region or country and are known only to a local expert. House wines in a good restaurant can often be excellent, at a very favorable cost.

Serving Wine

Wines are served in a very definite progression, from the lighter wines at the beginning of the meal toward the richer and more hearty ones with the subsequent courses. For example, you shouldn't drink a Macon after a Pommard, nor a Bordeaux after a Burgundy.

One drinks white wines and rosés very cold. Beaujolais should be chilled, Bordeaux at room temperature, Burgundy just a bit warmer than room temperature.

Sweet wines should be chilled and champagne iced (served and maintained in an ice bucket), but not frozen.

Extra-dry champagne (**brut**) is the only wine that can be served from one end of a meal to the other, and goes well with just about any dish. A meal usually ends with dessert, except for true wine lovers who would rather end the meal with cheese and sometimes nuts, in order to complement the flavor and aroma of a wine. In this case, it's the wine that becomes the dessert.

Serving Liqueurs

The ruddy liqueurs such as cognac and Armagnac are served in special small glasses whose bowls can be cradled in the palm of the hand, in order to transfer body heat to the liqueur, thus releasing its aroma. Fruity liqueurs of fruit based brandies (plum, raspberry, pear) are served chilled.

How to Say It: English to French

Numbers

1	one	un
2	two	deux
3	three	trois
4	four	quatre
5	five	cinq
6	six	six
7	seven	sept
8	eight	huit
9	nine	neuf
10	ten	dix
11	eleven	onze
12	twelve	douze
13	thirteen	treize
14	fourteen	quatorze
15	fifteen	quinze
16	sixteen	seize
17	seventeen	dix-sept
18	eighteen	dix-huit
19	nineteen	dix-neuf
20	twenty	vingt
21	twenty-one	vingt et un
22	twenty-two	vingt-deux
30	thirty	trente
40	forty	quarante
50	fifty	cinquante
60	sixty	soixante

70	seventy	soixante-dix
80	eighty	quatre-vingts
90	ninety	quatre-vingt-dix
100	one hundred	cent
101	one hundred one	cent un
102	one hundred two	cent deux
200	two hundred	deux cents
1,000	one thousand	mille
1,100	one thousand one hundred	mille cent
1,101	one thousand one hundred one	mille cent un
1,000,000	one million	un million
1,101,101	one million one hundred one thousand one hundred one	un million cent un mille cent un

Words and Phrases

AGAIN   encore
ALL   tout
ALL RIGHT   Ça va
ALSO   aussi
AS SOON AS POSSIBLE   Aussitôt que possible
ASHTRAY, PLEASE (AN)   Un cendrier, s'il vous plaît
ASK THE HEAD WAITER TO SEE ME HERE   Faites venir le maître d'hôtel ici
BACK   le dos
BAD   mauvais
BAKED   cuit au four
BAKED IN PARCHMENT   cuit au four en papillote
BARTENDER   le barman
BATHROOM   la salle de bain
BETTER   meilleur
BETTER THAN   meilleur que
BIG   grand

BOIL   bouillir
BOILED   à la coque
BOTTLE   une bouteille (la)
BRAISED   braisé
BREAKFAST   le petit déjeuner
CAN I HAVE...?   Puis-je avoir...?
CAN WE DINE NOW?   Pouvons-nous dîner maintenant?
CAN YOU HELP ME?   Pouvez-vous m'aider?
CHEAP   bon marché
CHECK   (un) le chèque
CHEERS!   santé!
CLOSE   fermer
COLD   froid
COME HERE   Venez ici
COME IN   Entrez
COULD WE HAVE SOME MORE?   Peut-on en avoir plus?
COVER CHARGE, MINIMUM   le couvert, le minimum
CUP   la tasse (une)
CUP OF COFFEE   une tasse de café
CURED   fumé/salé
DAY   le jour (un)
DELIGHTED   Enchanté
DIFFICULT   difficile
DINING ROOM   la salle à manger
DO YOU HAVE ANY...?   Avez-vous des...?
DO YOU SELL WINE BY THE GLASS?   Est-ce qu'on sert
   du vin au verre?
DO YOU UNDERSTAND?   Comprenez-vous?
DOES ANYONE SPEAK ENGLISH?   Est-ce que
   quelqu'un parle l'anglais?
DON'T MENTION IT   Je vous en prie
EARLY   tôt
EASY   facile
EAT   manger
EMERGENCY   une urgence/circonstance critique
EMPTY   vide
ENJOY YOUR MEAL   Bon appétit

ENOUGH   assez
EXCUSE ME   Excusez-moi
EXPENSIVE   cher
EYEGLASSES   des lunettes
FASTER   plus vite
FAT   gras, grasse
FEW   quelques
FIRE   du feu
FORK   une fourchette (la)
FREE   libre
FRIDAY   vendredi
FRONT (IN FRONT OF)   devant
FULL   plein
FULL-BODIED   un vin qui a une belle robe
FUNNY   amusant
GLASS   le verre (un)
GO AWAY!   Allez-vous-en!
GOOD   bon
GOOD AFTERNOON   Bonne après-midi
GOOD DAY   Bonjour
GOOD EVENING   Bonsoir
GOOD MORNING   Bon matin
GOOD NIGHT   Bonne nuit
GOOD-BYE   Au revoir
GREASE   la graisse
GREEN   vert, verte
HARD   dur
HAVE A GOOD MEAL   Bon appétit
HEADWAITER   le maître d'hôtel
HEART ATTACK   une crise cardiaque
HEAVY   lourd
HELLO   Salut
HERE   ici
HIGH   haut
HOSPITAL   l'hôpital (un)
HOT   chaud
HOT DISHES   des plats chauds

HOT FIRST COURSES   des entrées chaudes
HOT MAIN COURSES   des plats de résistance
HOW   comment
HOW ARE YOU? - NOT TOO BAD, THANK YOU - VERY
   WELL, THANK YOU   Comment allez-vous? Ça va,
   merci - Très bien, merci
HOW MANY?   Combien?
HOW MUCH IS IT?   Combien est-ce que c'est?
HOW MUCH WILL IT COST?   Combien est-ce que ça va
   coûter?
HUNGRY (I'M)   J'ai faim
HURRY   Dépêchez-vous
HURRY PLEASE   Dépêchez-vous, s'il vous plaît
I AM AN AMERICAN   Je suis un Américain
I AM HUNGRY   J'ai faim
I AM NOT IN A HURRY   Je ne suis pas pressé
I AM SORRY   Je suis désolé
I AM THIRSTY   J'ai soif
I AM WAITING FOR SOMEONE   J'attends quelqu'un
I DON'T KNOW   Je ne sais pas
I HAVE HAD ENOUGH, THANKS   Cela me suffit, merci
I HAVE LOST MY COAT   J'ai perdu mon manteau
I HAVE LOST MY MONEY   J'ai perdu ma monnaie
I HAVE LOST MY PASSPORT   J'ai perdu mon passeport
I KNOW   Je le sais
I LIKE THAT   J'aime ça
I SPEAK ONLY ENGLISH   Je parle seulement l'anglais
I'D LIKE...   Je voudrais...
I'LL TAKE THIS   Je le prendrais
I'M HUNGRY   J'ai faim
I'M IN A HURRY   Je suis pressé
I'M LOST   Je suis perdu
I'M SORRY   Pardon
IMMEDIATELY   tout de suite
IN   dans
IN THE AFTERNOON   pendant l'après-midi
IN THE EVENING   au soir (le)_

IN THE MORNING   au matin (le)
INSTEAD   au lieu de
IT DOESN'T MATTER   Ça ne fait rien
IT IS   C'est
IT IS GOOD   C'est bon
IT IS VERY GOOD   C'est très bon
KNIFE   le couteau (un)
KOSHER   cacher (cachère)
LADIES' ROOM   toilette de dames
LADIES   Mesdames
LARGE SPOON   une grande cuillère
LAST   dernier
LAST NIGHT   hier soir
LATE   tard
LATER   plus tard
LAVATORY   les toilettes
LEAN   maigre
LEFT   gauche
LIGHT   léger
LISTEN!   Ecoutez!
LOW   bas
MATCH   une allumette
MAY I HAVE THE MENU?   Puis-je avoir le menu?
MAY I HAVE THIS?   Puis-je avoir ceci?
MEAL   le repas (un)
MEAL SERVED QUICKLY   un repas rapide
MEDIUM   à point
MEDIUM RARE   saignant
MEN'S   des hommes/des messieurs
MEN'S ROOM   toilette pour hommes
MENU   un menu
MID-MORNING SNACK   un en-cas matinal
MIDNIGHT   minuit
MONDAY   lundi
MORE   en plus
MY NAME IS...   Je m'appelle...
NAPKIN   une serviette

NEAR près
NEED un besoin (le)
NEW nouveau
NEXT prochain
NIGHT la nuit (une)
NO non
NOON midi
NOTHING MORE, THANKS Rien de plus, merci
NOW maintenant
OCCUPIED occupé
OLD vieux
ON sur
OPEN ouvert
PASTRY CART le plateau de pâtisseries
PAY payer
PEPPER MILL moulin à poivre
PERHAPS peut-être
PHARMACY pharmacie
PIECE un morceau
PITCHER une cruche
PLACE SETTING un couvert
PLATE une assiette
PLEASE s'il vous plaît
PLEASE BRING ME ANOTHER FORK Apportez-moi
  une autre fourchette, s'il vous plaît
POACHED poché
PREFER préférer
PREPARED AT THE TABLE préparé à la table
RARE saignant
RAW bleu
RED WINE du vin rouge (un)
REQUEST une demande (la)
RESTAURANT un restaurant (le)
RIGHT à droite
RIGHT (CORRECT) c'est juste (correct)
ROAST un rôti (le)
SATURDAY samedi

SAUTÉED   sauté
SEASONING   l'assaisonnement
SEE YOU LATER   à tout à l'heure
SEE YOU SOON   à bientôt
SERIOUS   grave
SEVERAL   plusieurs
SHUT   fermé
SLICE OF (A)   une tranche de...
SMALL   petit
SMALL BOTTLE OF...   une petite bouteille de...
SMOKED   fumé
SNACK   un goûter
SOFT   mou, molle
SOON   bientôt
SOUP SPOON   une cuillère à soupe
SPECTACLES   des lunettes
SPICY SAUCE   une sauce épicée
SPOON   une cuillère (la)
STEAMED   cuit à la vapeur
STEWED   à l'étuvée
STUPID   stupide
SUNDAY   dimanche
SUPPER   le souper (un)
SWEET   l'entremets (des)
TABLE   une table (la)
TABLESPOON   une grande cuillère (la)
TEASPOON   une petite cuillère
TELEPHONE   un téléphone
THANK YOU   merci
THANKS VERY MUCH   Merci beaucoup
THE DAY BEFORE YESTERDAY   avant-hier
THERE   là
THERE HAS BEEN AN ACCIDENT   Il y a eu un accident
THIRSTY (I'M)   J'ai soif
THURSDAY   jeudi
TOASTED   grillé

TODAY aujourd'hui
TOILET la toilette (une)
TOILET FOR LADIES toilettes pour dames
TOILET FOR MEN toilettes pour messieurs
TOMORROW demain
TONIGHT ce soir
TOO aussi
TOOTHPICK un cure-dent (le)
TUESDAY mardi
UGLY laid
VERY DRY très sec
VERY GOOD! Très bien!
WAIT A MOMENT Attendez un moment
WAITER! Garçon!
WAITRESS! Mademoiselle!
WE WOULD LIKE A BOTTLE OF GOOD LOCAL WINE
　Nous voudrions une bonne bouteille de vin du pays
WEDNESDAY mercredi
WELL-DONE bien cuit
WHAT A PITY! Quel dommage!
WHAT DO YOU WANT? Que voulez-vous?
WHAT'S THE MATTER? Qu'est-ce qu'il y a?
WHAT? Quoi?
WHEN? Quand?
WHERE IS THE TOILET? Où sont les toilettes?
WHERE? Où?
WHITE WINE du vin blanc (le)
WHO? Qui?
WHY NOT? Pourquoi pas?
WHY? Pourquoi?
WILD sauvage
WINE GLASS un verre à vin
WINE LIST la carte des vins
WITH avec
WITHOUT sans
WORSE pire

YES   oui
YESTERDAY   hier
YOU ARE WELCOME   De rien

Food and Drink

ALMOND   une amande
ANCHOVIES   des anchois
APPETIZER   un hors-d'oeuvre
APPLE   une pomme (des pommes)
APPLESAUCE   une purée de pommes
APRICOT   un abricot
ARTICHOKE   un artichaut
ASPARAGUS   des asperges
ASSORTED CHEESES   des fromages assortis
AVOCADOS   des avocats
BACON   du lard
BACON AND EGGS   des oeufs au lard
BANANA   une banane
BASKET OF FRUIT   un panier de fruits
BEANS   des haricots
BEEF   du boeuf
BEEFSTEAK   du bifteck
BEER   de la bière
BEER BOTTLED   une bouteille de bière
BEER DARK   de la bière brune
BEER DRAFT   de la bière à la pression
BEER LIGHT   de la bière blonde
BISCUITS   des biscuits
BLACK COFFEE   du café noir
BLACK OLIVES   des olives noires
BOILED EGG, HARD   un oeuf à la coque dur
BOILED EGG, MEDIUM   un oeuf à la coque moyen
BOILED EGG, SOFT   un oeuf à la coque mollet
BRANDY   du cognac
BREAD   du pain
BREAKFAST SAUSAGE   de la saucisse

BROCCOLI   du brocoli
BURGUNDY   du vin de Bourgogne
BUTTER   du beurre
CABBAGE   du chou (un)
CAKE   un gâteau
CANDY   des bonbons
CARAFE OF LOCAL RED WINE PLEASE   Une carafe de
   vin rouge du pays, s'il vous plaît
CARP   de la carpe
CARROTS   des carottes
CAULIFLOWER   du chou-fleur
CELERY   du celéri
CEREAL COLD   des céréales froides
CEREAL HOT   des céréales chaudes
CHAMPAGNE   du champagne
CHEESE   du fromage
CHERRIES   des cerises
CHICKEN   du poulet
CHICKEN FRICASSEE   du poulet fricassé
CHICKEN FRIED   du poulet frit
CHICKEN ROAST   du poulet rôti
CHICKEN SOUP   du bouillon de poulet
CHIPS   des pommes frites
CHOCOLATE   du chocolat
CHOCOLATE BAR   une plaque de chocolat
CHOP   une côtelette
CHOPPED STEAK   de la viande hachée
CLAMS   des palourdes
COCKTAIL   un cocktail
COD   du cabillaud
COFFEE   du café
COFFEE AMERICAN FILTERED   du café américain filtré
COFFEE BLACK   du café noir
COFFEE DECAFFEINATED   café décaféiné
COFFEE ICED   café glacé
COFFEE INSTANT   café soluble
COFFEE WITH CREAM   du café avec crème

COFFEE WITH HOT MILK   du café au lait chaud
COFFEE, ROLLS, BUTTER   du café, des petits pain et du beurre
COGNAC   du Cognac
COLD MILK   du lait froid
CONTINENTAL BREAKFAST   du café complet
COOKIES   des petits gâteaux secs
CORN   du maïs
CRABS   des crabes
CRAYFISH   des écrevisses
CREAM   de la crème
CUCUMBER   un concombre
CUSTARD   de la crème
DESSERT   un dessert
DINNER   le dîner
DRINK   une boisson
DRY   sec
DUCK   du canard
EAT   manger
EEL   des anguilles
EGGS   des oeufs
EGGS BOILED   des oeufs à la coque
EGGS BOILED FIRM   des oeufs solides
EGGS BOILED HARD   des oeufs durs
EGGS BOILED SOFT   des oeufs tendres
EGGS FRIED   des oeufs frits sur le plat
EGGS FRIED OVER   des oeufs frits retournés
EGGS FRIED UP   des oeufs frits haut
EGGS FRIED WITH BACON   des oeufs grillés avec du lard
EGGS FRIED WITH HAM   des oeufs grillés avec du jambon
EGGS FRIED WITH POTATOES   des oeufs grillés avec des pommes de terre
EGGS FRIED WITH SAUSAGE   des oeufs grillés avec de la saucisse
EGGS POACHED   des oeufs pochés
EGGS POACHED FIRM   des oeufs pochés durs
EGGS POACHED SOFT   des oeufs pochés tendres

EGGS SCRAMBLED   des oeufs brouillés
EGGS SCRAMBLED WITH BACON   des oeufs brouillés
    au lard
EGGS SCRAMBLED WITH HAM   des oeufs brouillés au
    jambon
EGGS SCRAMBLED WITH POTATOES   des oeufs
    brouillés avec des pommes de terre
EGGS SCRAMBLED WITH SAUSAGE   des oeufs
    brouillés à la saucisse
ESPRESSO BLACK   un café express
ESPRESSO WEAK   allongé
ESPRESSO WITH MILK   café au lait
FISH   du poisson
FRENCH ROLLS   des petits pains
FRIED   frit; sur le plat
FRIED EGGS   des oeufs sur le plat
FRIED POTATOES   des frites
FROG LEGS   des cuisses de grenouilles
FRUIT   du fruit
FRUIT COMPOTE   de la compote de fruits
FRUIT DRINK   un jus de fruits
FRUIT JUICE   un jus de fruits
FRUIT SALAD   la macédoine de fruits
FULL-BODIED   Un vin qui a une belle robe
GAME   du gibier
GARLIC   de l'ail
GIN   du gin
GIN AND TONIC   un gin-tonique
GLASS OF MILK   un verre de lait
GLASS OF WATER   un verre d'eau
GLASS OF WINE   un verre de vin
GOOSE   une oie
GOOSE LIVER PASTE   un pâté de foie gras
GRAPE   un raisin
GRAPEFRUIT   du pamplemousse
GRAPEFRUIT JUICE   un jus de pamplemousse
GRAVY   une sauce

GREEN BEANS   des haricots verts
GREEN OLIVES   des olives vertes
GREEN PEPPER   un poivron vert
GREEN SALAD   une salade verte
GREEN VEGETABLES   des légumes verts
HADDOCK   un aiglefin
HALIBUT   un flétan
HAM   du jambon
HEN   de la poule
HERRING   du hareng
HONEY   du miel
HOT CHOCOLATE   du chocolat chaud
HOT MILK   du lait chaud
HOT WATER   de l'eau chaude
ICE   de la glace
ICE CUBES   des glaçons
ICE WATER   de l'eau glacée
ICE CREAM   une glace
JAM   de la confiture
JUICE   du jus
KETCHUP   du ketchup
KIDNEYS   des rognons
LAMB   de l'agneau
LAMB CHOPS   des côtelettes d'agneau
LEMON   du citron
LEMONADE   de la citronnade
LETTUCE   de la laitue
LIMA BEANS   des haricots de Lima
LIQUEUR   une liqueur
LIVER   du foie
LOBSTER   un homard
MACKEREL   du maquereau
MARMALADE   de la confiture d'oranges
MASHED POTATOES   de la purée de pommes de terre
MAYONNAISE   de la mayonnaise
MEAT   de la viande
MEATBALLS   des boulettes de viande

MILK   du lait
MINERAL WATER   de l'eau minérale
MIXED SALAD   de la salade panachée
MUSHROOMS   des champignons
MUSSELS   des moules
MUSTARD   de la moutarde
MUTTON   du mouton
NOODLES   des nouilles
NUT   une noix
OATMEAL   de la bouillie d'avoine
OIL   de l'huile
OLIVE   de l'olive
OLIVE OIL   de l'huile d'olive
OMELET   une omelette
ONION   un oignon
ORANGE   de l'orange
ORANGE JUICE   du jus d'orange
OYSTER   des huîtres
PANCAKES   des crêpes
PARSLEY   du persil
PASTRY   de la pâtisserie
PEACH   une pêche
PEANUTS   des cacahouètes
PEAR   une poire
PEAS   des petits pois
PEPPER   du poivre
PIE   une tarte
PIGEON   un pigeon
PIKE   du brochet
PINEAPPLE   de l'ananas
PLUM   une prune
PORK   du porc
PORK CHOPS   des côtelettes de porc
PORT   un porto
POTATO   une pomme de terre
POTATO SALAD   une salade de pommes de terre
POTATOES BOILED   des pommes de terre bouillies

POTATOES FRIED   des frites
POTATOES MASHED   une purée de pommes de terre
POULTRY   du poulet
PRAWNS   des langoustines
PRUNES   des prunes
RABBIT   du lapin
RADISHES   des radis
RASPBERRIES   des framboises
RED CABBAGE   du chou rouge
RED WINE   du vin rouge (un)
RICE   du riz
ROAST BEEF   du rosbif
ROAST CHICKEN   du poulet rôti
ROAST PORK   du rôti de porc
ROAST VEAL   du rôti de veau
ROLLS   des petits pains
ROSÉ WINE   du vin rosé
RUM   du rhum
SACCHARIN   de la saccharine
SALAD   de la salade
SALAD DRESSING   de la vinaigrette
SALAMI   du saucisson
SALMON   du saumon
SALT   du sel
SANDWICH   un sandwich
SAUCE   de la sauce
SAUERKRAUT   de la choucroute
SAUSAGE   une saucisse
SCOTCH   un scotch
SCRAMBLED EGGS   des oeufs brouillés
SEA BASS   loup de mer
SEAFOOD   des fruits de mer
SHARK   un requin
SHERRY   du sherry
SHRIMP   des crevettes
SHRIMP COCKTAIL   du cocktail de crevettes
SNAILS   des escargots

SODA   du soda
SOFT DRINKS   sodas/boissons sans alcool
SOUP   du potage
SPAGHETTI   du spaghetti
SPARKLING (WATER)   gazeuse; (WINE)   mousseux
SPINACH   des épinards
SQUID   du calmar
STEAK   un bifteck
STEW   du ragoût
STRAWBERRIES   des fraises
SUGAR   du sucre
SWEETS   des bonbons
TEA   du thé
TEA WITH CREAM   du thé à la crème
TEA WITH LEMON   du thé au citron
TOAST   du pain grillé
TOMATO   une tomate
TOMATO SAUCE   de la sauce de tomate
TONGUE   une langue
TROUT   de la truite
TRUFFLE   une truffe
TUNA   du thon
TURKEY   une dinde
VANILLA   de la vanille
VEAL   du veau
VEGETABLE   un légume
VEGETABLE SOUP   une soupe de légumes
VERMOUTH   du vermouth
VERY DRY   très sec
VINEGAR   du vinaigre
VODKA   une vodka
WATER   de l'eau
WATERMELON   une pastèque
WHIPPED CREAM   de la crème
WHISKEY   du whisky
WHISKEY AND SODA   du whisky et du soda
WHITE WINE   du vin blanc (le)

WINE   du vin
WINE LOCAL RED   un vin rouge du pays
WINE LOCAL WHITE   un vin blanc du pays
WINE RED   du vin rouge
WINE SPARKLING   du vin mousseux
WINE VERY DRY   du vin très sec
WINE VERY FULL BODIED   du vin qui a une belle robe
WINE WHITE   du vin blanc
YOGURT   du yaourt

In the Restaurant: To Order or Make Requests

A TABLE BY THE WINDOW PLEASE   Une table près de la fenêtre, s'il vous plaît
A TABLE FOR THREE PLEASE   Une table pour trois, s'il vous plaît
A TABLE OUTSIDE PLEASE   Une table dehors, s'il vous plaît
ANOTHER CHAIR   une chaise de plus
ASHTRAY, PLEASE (AN)   Un cendrier, s'il vous plaît
ASK THE HEADWAITER TO SEE ME HERE   Faites venir le maître d'hôtel
AT WHAT TIMES ARE MEALS SERVED?   A quelle heure servez-vous les repas?
BATHROOM   la salle de bain
BILL OR CHECK PLEASE   L'addition s'il vous plaît
BREAKFAST   le petit déjeuner
BRING ME THE MENU PLEASE   Apportez-moi le menu, s'il vous plaît
BRING ME THE WINE LIST PLEASE   Apportez-moi la carte des vins s'il vous plaît
BRING THE CHECK, PLEASE   Apportez l'addition, s'il vous plaît
BRING US SOME COFFEE NOW, PLEASE   Apportez-nous du café maintenant, s'il vous plaît
CAN I HAVE...?   Puis-je avoir...?

Have you decided? Avez-vous choisi?

CAN WE DINE NOW?   Pouvons-nous dîner maintenant?

CAN YOU RECOMMEND A GOOD RESTAURANT?
Connaissez-vous un bon restaurant, s'il vous plaît?

CAN YOU RECOMMEND A GOOD RESTAURANT, NOT
TOO EXPENSIVE?   Connaissez-vous un bon restaurant, pas trop cher?

CARAFE OF LOCAL RED WINE PLEASE   Une carafe de vin rouge du pays s'il vous plaît

CARAFE OF LOCAL WHITE WINE PLEASE   Une carafe de vin blanc du pays, s'il vous plaît

CHECK   (un) le chèque

COULD WE HAVE SOME MORE...?   Peut-on en avoir plus...?

CUP   la tasse (une)

CUP OF COFFEE   une tasse de café

DINING ROOM   la salle à manger

DO YOU ACCEPT AMERICAN MONEY?   Acceptez-vous de la monnaie américaine?

DO YOU ACCEPT AMERICAN EXPRESS CARDS?
Acceptez-vous la carte American Express?

DO YOU ACCEPT DINERS CARD?   Acceptez-vous la carte Diners?

DO YOU ACCEPT MASTER CARD?   Acceptez-vous la carte Master?

DO YOU ACCEPT VISA CARDS?   Acceptez-vous la carte Visa?

DO YOU HAVE A DISH OF THE DAY?   Avez-vous un plat du jour?

DO YOU HAVE ANY...?   Avez-vous des...?

DO YOU SELL WINE BY THE GLASS?   Est-ce qu'on sert du vin au verre?

DO YOU UNDERSTAND?   Comprenez-vous?

FORK   une fourchette (la)

GLASS OF ... PLEASE   Un verre de ... s'il vous plaît

GLASS OF BEER   Un verre de bière

GLASS OF LIQUEUR   Un verre de liqueur

GRILLED   grillé

HAVE YOU A SET MENU?   Avez-vous un menu à prix fixe?

HAVE YOU A TABLE FOR ... PEOPLE   Avez-vous une
    table pour ... personnes?

HAVE YOU ANY ...   Avez-vous des ...

HAVE YOU COMPLETE DINNERS?   Avez-vous des
    dîners complets?

HOT FIRST COURSES   des entrées chaudes

HOT MAIN COURSES   des plats de résistance

HOTTER   plus chaud

HOW MANY?   Combien?

I AM HUNGRY   J'ai faim

I AM IN A HURRY   Je suis pressé

I AM THIRSTY   J'ai soif

I HAVE HAD ENOUGH, THANKS   Cela me suffit merci

I LIKE THAT   J'aime ça

I LIKE THE MEAT RARE   J'aime la viande saignante

I LIKE THE MEAT WELL DONE   J'aime la viande bien
    cuite

I SHOULD LIKE TO SEE THE HEADWAITER   Je
    voudrais voir le maître d'hôtel

I WANT   Je veux

I WANT SOMETHING SIMPLE. NOT TOO SPICY   Je
    veux quelque chose de simple. Pas trop épicé

I WOULD LIKE A BOTTLE OF WINE   Je voudrais une
    bouteille de vin

I WOULD LIKE A GLASS OF RED WINE   Je voudrais un
    verre de vin rouge

I WOULD LIKE A GLASS OF WHITE WINE   Je voudrais
    un verre de vin blanc

I WOULD LIKE A GLASS OF WINE   Je voudrai un verre
    de vin

I'D LIKE A DESSERT PLEASE   Je prendrais un dessert,
    s'il vous plaît

I'D LIKE AN APERITIF   Je voudrais un apéritif

I'D LIKE AN APPETIZER   Je voudrais une entrée

I'D LIKE SOME BEEF   Je voudrais du boeuf

I'D LIKE SOME FISH   Je voudrais du poisson

I'D LIKE SOME LAMB   Je voudrais de l'agneau
I'D LIKE SOME PORK   Je voudrais du porc
I'D LIKE SOME VEAL   Je voudrais du veau
I'D LIKE THE MEAT MEDIUM   Je voudrais la viande à
   point
I'D LIKE TO RESERVE A TABLE FOR FOUR AT ...   Je
   voudrais réserver une table pour quatre pour ... heures
I'D LIKE...   Je voudrais...
I'LL TAKE THIS   Je le prendrais
I'M HUNGRY   J'ai faim
IS EVERYTHING INCLUDED?   Est-ce que tout y est
   compris?
KNIFE   le couteau (un)
KOSHER   cacher (cachère)
LADIES   Mesdames
LARGE SPOON   une grande cuillère
LAVATORY   les toilettes
LEAN   maigre
LOCAL RED WINE   du vin rouge du pays
LOCAL WHITE WINE   du vin blanc du pays
LOCAL WINE   du vin du pays
MAY I CHANGE THIS?   Puis-je changer ceci?
MAY I HAVE THE MENU?   Puis-je avoir le menu?
MAY I HAVE THE WINE LIST?   Puis-je avoir la carte des
   vins?
MAY I HAVE THIS?   Puis-je avoir ceci?
MEAL SERVED QUICKLY   un repas rapide
MEDIUM   à point
MEDIUM RARE   saignant
MEN'S   des hommes/des messieurs
MENU   un menu
MENU PLEASE   Un menu s'il vous plaît
MID MORNING SNACK   un en-cas matinal
MORE BEER, PLEASE   Plus de bière, s'il vous plaît
MORE BREAD, PLEASE   Plus de pain, s'il vous plaît
MORE COFFEE PLEASE   Plus de café, s'il vous plaît
MORE PLEASE   Encore, s'il vous plaît

MORE WATER, PLEASE   Encore de l'eau, s'il vous plaît
NAPKIN   une serviette
NO SAUCE, PLEASE   Pas de sauce, s'il vous plaît
ON THE ROCKS   avec des glaçons
PASTRY CART   Le plateau de pâtisseries
PEPPER MILL   un moulin à poivre
PLATE   une assiette
PLEASE BRING ME ANOTHER FORK   Apportez-moi
   une autre fourchette, s'il vous plaît
PLEASE SERVE US QUICKLY   Servez-nous vite, s'il vous plaît
PREFER   préférer
RARE   saignant
SALT   du sel
SEASONING   l'assaisonnement
SLICE OF (A)   Une tranche de...
SOME COFFEE, PLEASE   Du café, s'il vous plaît
SOMETHING LIGHT, PLEASE   Quelque chose de léger,
   s'il vous plaît
SOUP SPOON   une cuillère à soupe
SPICY SAUCE   une sauce épicée
SPOON   une cuillère (la)
SUGAR   du sucre
TABLE   une table (la)
TABLE FOR TWO, PLEASE   Deux couverts, s'il vous plaît
TABLESPOON   une grande cuillère (la)
TAKE IT AWAY, PLEASE   Emportez-le, s'il vous plaît
TEASPOON   une petite cuillère
TOASTED   grillé
TOILET FOR LADIES   toilettes pour dames
TOILET FOR MEN   toilettes pour messieurs
TOOTHPICK   un cure-dent (le)
WE SHOULD LIKE A BOTTLE OF DRY WINE   Nous
   voudrions une bouteille de vin sec
WE SHOULD LIKE A BOTTLE OF RED WINE   Nous
   voudrions une bouteille de vin rouge
WE SHOULD LIKE A BOTTLE OF SWEET WINE   Nous
   voudrions une bouteille de vin doux

WE SHOULD LIKE A BOTTLE OF WHITE WINE   Nous
   voudrions une bouteille de vin blanc
WE WOULD LIKE A BOTTLE OF GOOD LOCAL WINE
   Nous voudrions une bonne bouteille de vin du pays
WELL-DONE   bien cuit
WHAT DO YOU HAVE FOR DESSERT?   Qu'avez-vous
   comme dessert?
WHAT DO YOU RECOMMEND?   Que me recommandez-
   vous?
WHAT IS THAT?/IT'S A...   Qu'est-ce que c'est? C'est un...
WHAT IS THE SPECIALTY OF THE HOUSE?   Quelle est
   la spécialité de la maison?
WHAT IS THE TIME?   Quelle heure est-il?
WHAT IS THIS?   Qu'est-ce que c'est?
WHAT KINDS OF SEAFOOD DO YOU HAVE?   Quel
   genre de fruits de mer servez-vous?
WHAT SALADS DO YOU HAVE?   Quelles salades avez-
   vous?
WHAT WINE DO YOU RECOMMEND?   Quel vin
   recommandez-vous?
WHERE IS THE TOILET?   Où sont les toilettes?
WINE GLASS   un verre à vin
WINE LIST   la carte des vins
WINE LIST PLEASE   La carte des vins, s'il vous plaît
WINE LOCAL RED   un vin rouge du pays
WINE LOCAL WHITE   un vin blanc du pays
WINE VERY FULL BODIED   du vin qui a une belle robe
WINE WHAT DO YOU RECOMMEND?   Quel vin
   recommandez-vous?
WITH SELTZER WATER   à l'eau de Seltz
WITHOUT ICE   sans glaçons

Problems

DIRTY   sale
I AM IN A HURRY   Je suis pressé
I AM LOST   Je suis perdu

I ASKED FOR ...   J'ai demandé ...
I DID NOT ORDER THIS   Je n'ai pas commandé cela
I DO NOT UNDERSTAND   Je ne comprends pas
I DON'T LIKE THAT   Je n'aime pas ça
I HAVE LOST MY COAT   J'ai perdu mon manteau
I HAVE LOST MY MONEY   J'ai perdu mon argent
I HAVE LOST MY PASSPORT   J'ai perdu mon passeport
I SHOULD LIKE TO SEE THE HEADWAITER   Je
    voudrais voir le maître d'hôtel
I THINK THERE IS A MISTAKE HERE   Je crois qu'il y a
    une erreur ici
I'M IN A HURRY   Je suis pressé
I'M LOST   Je suis perdu
IS THERE ANYONE HERE WHO KNOWS FIRST AID?
    Y a-t-il quelqu'un qui connaît les premiers secours ici?
IT DOES NOT TASTE RIGHT   Le goût n'est pas bon
IT IS NOT GOOD   Ce n'est pas bon
IT ISN'T HOT ENOUGH   Ce n'est pas assez chaud
MAY I CHANGE THIS?   Puis-je changer ceci?
STOP!   Arrêtez-vous!
THAT IS BAD   C'est mauvais
THE BILL IS INCORRECT   Il y a une erreur dans l'addition
THE FISH IS BAD   Le poisson n'est pas bon
THE MEAT IS BAD   La viande n'est pas bonne
THE MEAT IS OVERDONE   La viande est trop cuite
THE MEAT IS TOO RARE   La viande est trop saignante
THE MEAT IS TOO TOUGH   La viande est trop dure
THE MEAT IS UNDERDONE   La viande n'est pas assez
    cuite
THE SOUP IS COLD   Le potage est froid
THE WINE IS CORKED   Ce vin sent le bouchon
THIS IS COLD   C'est froid
THIS IS NOT CLEAN   Ce n'est pas propre
THIS IS NOT COOKED   Ce n'est pas cuit
THIS IS NOT WHAT I ORDERED   Ce n'est pas ce que j'ai
    commandé
THIS IS OVERCOOKED   C'est trop cuit

THIS IS TOO SOUR   C'est trop amer
THIS IS TOO SWEET   C'est trop sucré
THIS IS TOO TOUGH   C'est trop dur
THIS IS UNDERCOOKED   Ce n'est pas assez cuit
TOO BAD!   Tant pis!
TOO MUCH   trop
WE ARE IN A HURRY   Nous sommes pressés
WRONG   faux

To Pay

BILL   l'addition
BILL OR CHECK PLEASE   L'addition s'il vous plaît
BRING THE CHECK, PLEASE   Apportez l'addition, s'il
   vous plaît
CHECK   (un) le chèque
COVER CHARGE, MINIMUM   Le couvert, le minimum
DO YOU ACCEPT AMERICAN MONEY?   Acceptez-vous
   de la monnaie américaine?
DO YOU ACCEPT AMERICAN EXPRESS CARDS?
   Acceptez-vous la carte American Express?
DO YOU ACCEPT DINERS CARD?   Acceptez-vous la
   carte Diners?
DO YOU ACCEPT MASTER CARD?   Acceptez-vous la
   carte Master?
DO YOU ACCEPT VISA CARDS?   Acceptez-vous la carte
   Visa?
I THINK THERE IS A MISTAKE HERE   Je crois qu'il y a
   une erreur ici
IS EVERYTHING INCLUDED?   Est-ce que tout y est
   compris?
IS THE DRINK INCLUDED?   Boisson comprise?
IS THE SERVICE CHARGE INCLUDED?   Le service, est-il
   compris?
IS THE TIP INCLUDED?   Le pourboire, est-il compris?
IT IS VERY EXPENSIVE   C'est très cher
MAY WE HAVE THE BILL, PLEASE   L'addition, s'il vous plaît

PAY   payer
SERVICE INCLUDED   service compris
SERVICE NOT INCLUDED   service non compris
THE BILL IS INCORRECT   Il y a une erreur dans
l'addition
THE CHECK PLEASE   L'addition, s'il vous plaît
THERE IS A MISTAKE IN THE BILL   Il y a une erreur
dans l'addition

Doctor, Dentist, Emergency

CALL A DOCTOR   Appelez un médecin
CALL AN AMBULANCE   Appelez une ambulance
CAN YOU GET ME A DOCTOR WHO SPEAKS ENGLISH?
IT'S URGENT!   Pouvez-vous m'appeler un médecin
qui parle l'anglais? C'est urgent!
CAN YOU RECOMMEND A GOOD DENTIST?   Pouvez-
vous recommander un bon dentiste?
DENTIST   un dentiste (le)
DENTIST: JUST FIX IT TEMPORARILY   Arranger-le
temporairement
DOES ANYONE SPEAK ENGLISH?   Est-ce que
quelqu'un parle l'anglais?
EMERGENCY   une urgence/circonstance critique
FIRE!   Au feu!
HEART ATTACK   une crise cardiaque
HELP!   Au secours!
HOSPITAL   l'hôpital (un)
I AM LOST   Je suis perdu
I FEEL SICK   Je me sens malade
I HAVE A TOOTHACHE   J'ai un mal de dents
IS THERE A DOCTOR HERE?   Y a-t-il un médecin ici?
IS THERE A DOCTOR WHO SPEAKS ENGLISH?   Y a-t-il
un médecin qui parle l'anglais?
IS THERE ANYONE HERE WHO KNOWS FIRST AID?
Y a-t-il quelqu'un qui connaît les premiers secours ici?
IT HURTS HERE   Ça me fait mal ici

PHARMACY   une pharmacie
THERE HAS BEEN AN ACCIDENT   Il y a eu un accident
WHEN CAN HE COME?   Quant peut-il venir?

Telephone/Taxi

ASK HIM/HER TO RING ME AT..., PLEASE   Demandez-lui de me rappeler à..., s'il vous plaît
CAN I DIAL DIRECT?   Puis-je téléphoner par l'automatique?
CAN YOU HELP ME GET THIS NUMBER?   Pouvez-vous m'aider à obtenir ce numéro?
DO I NEED TELEPHONE TOKENS?   Est-ce qui j'ai besoin de jetons pour le téléphone?
DO YOU SPEAK ENGLISH?   Parlez-vous l'anglais?
EXTENSION NUMBER .... PLEASE   Poste numéro, s'il vous plaît
GIVE ME THE LONG DISTANCE OPERATOR   Donnez-moi l'Inter
HOW MUCH IS A TELEPHONE CALL TO ...   Combien coûte un coup de fil à ...
I HAVE BEEN CUT OFF   La communication a été coupée
I WANT A LONG DISTANCE CALL ...   Je veux un coup de fil inter
I WANT NUMBER ... PLEASE   Je veux le numéro ... s'il vous plaît
I WANT TO MAKE A LOCAL CALL, NUMBER...   Donnez-moi la ville, numéro...
I WANT TO MAKE A PERSON-TO-PERSON CALL TO...   Je veux appeler avec préavis à...
I WANT TO MAKE A REVERSE CHARGE CALL TO....   Je veux téléphoner en p.c.v. à...
I WOULD LIKE A TELEPHONE TOKEN   Je voudrais un jeton pour le téléphone
I WOULD LIKE TO TELEPHONE....   Je voudrais téléphoner
MAY I SPEAK TO ....   Puis-je parler à ...
MAY I USE YOUR PHONE?   Puis-je utiliser votre téléphone?

MY NUMBER IS....   Mon numéro est ....

OCCUPIED   occupé

OPERATOR   un opérateur/une opératrice

PLEASE CALL A TAXI FOR ME   Veuillez m'appeler un taxi

PLEASE GET ME A TAXI   Appelez-moi un taxi, s'il vous plaît

PLEASE GIVE ME TWO TOKENS FOR THE PHONE   Donnez-moi deux jetons pour le téléphone, s'il vous plaît

PLEASE RECONNECT ME   Veuillez me rétablir

PLEASE SPEAK MORE SLOWLY   Parlez plus lentement s'il vous plaît

REPEAT PLEASE   Répétez, s'il vous plaît

SPEAKING IS ....   Qui parle est ...

TAXI   un taxi

TELEPHONE   un téléphone

TELL HIM THAT...'PHONED   Dites-lui que ... a téléphoné

THIS 'PHONE IS NOT WORKING   Cet appareil ne fonctionne pas

TOKENS   des jetons

WHAT COIN DO I PUT IN?   Je mets quelle pièce de monnaie dedans?

WHAT IS THE TELEPHONE NUMBER?   Quel est le numéro du téléphone?

WHERE IS THE TELEPHONE BOOK?   Où est l'annuaire?

WHERE'S THE TELEPHONE?   Où se trouve le téléphone?

WILL YOU TELEPHONE FOR ME?   Pouvez-vous bien téléphoner pour moi?

3

How to Understand It: French to English

Appetizers

AMUSE-GUEULE   appetizer
ANCHOÏADE   mashed anchovies on toast
ANCHOIS   anchovy
ANGES CHEVAL   grilled oysters with bacon
ANGUILLE FUMÉE   smoked eel
ARCACHON, HUÎTRE D'   oyster with a strong flavor
ARTICHAUT À LA VINAIGRETTE   artichoke with oil and vinegar dressing
ASPERGES D'ARGENTEUIL   best white asparagus
ASSIETTE ANGLAISE   platter of assorted cold cuts or cold meats
ASSIETTE CHARCUTERIE   plate of dried sausage and pâté
ASSIETTE DE CRUDITÉS   plate of raw vegetables with oil and vinegar
ASSIETTE DE VIANDES FROIDES   cold cuts of meat
ASSIETTE SALAMI   plate of various salamis
ATHÉRINE   fried smelt
AUBERGINE AU TOMATE   eggplant with tomato
BARQUETTE   pastry shell with various fillings
BARQUETTE ÉCOSSAISE   pastry shell with smoked salmon
BARQUETTE OSTENDAISE   pastry shells with creamed oysters
BATELIÈRE   pastry shells with seafood filling

BEIGNETS DE POISSON   miniature fish balls
BEIGNETS NIÇOIS   batter fried pieces of tunafish
BELONS   oysters
BELONS, DEMI-DOUZAINE DE   a half dozen oysters
BELONS, DOUZAINE DE   a dozen oysters
BELUGA   caviar
BEURSAUDES   bacon or pork fried, then baked
BOUCHÉE   individual puff pastry shells
BOUCHÉE À LA FINANCIÈRE   chicken and lambs'
   brains in creamy, sherry sauce
BOUCHÉE À LA REINE   pastry shells with mushrooms,
   tongue and chicken
BOUCHÉE AU FROMAGE   pastry shell with cheese
BOUFFI   smoked kipper
BRISOLETTE   a very small cocktail appetizer or hors
   d'oeuvre
BROCHETTE JURASSIENNE   pieces of cheese wrapped
   in ham and fried
BUFFET FROID   dishes served cold from a buffet
CAGOUILLES VIGNERONNE   snails cooked in white wine
CANAPÉS   toasted bread with a variety of garnishes
CANAPÉS À LA CRÈME DE FROMAGE   cream cheese
   on toast
CANAPÉS CREVETTES   shrimp canapes
CAPRES   capers
CAPUCINE MUSCOVITE   appetizer of shrimp and egg
   yolks on toast
CARGOLADE   snails
CARPE AU JUIF   boiled carp served cold in aspic
CAVIAR   sturgeon eggs
CAVIAR AUBERGINE   cold eggplant puree with fish eggs
CAVIAR BLANC   mullet eggs
CAVIAR FRAIS   fresh fish eggs
CAVIAR MALOSSIL   fish eggs, lightly salted
CAVIAR NIÇOIS   anchovies, oil, fish eggs, usually served
   on toast
CAVOUR   mushrooms stuffed with chicken liver

CÈPES À LA BORDELAISE   mushrooms sautéed in oil

CHAMPIGNONS À LA GRECQUE   cold mushrooms cooked in lemon juice and olive oil

CHAMPIGNONS FARCIS   mushrooms stuffed with butter, cream, Swiss cheese

CHAMPIGNONS FARCIS D'ÉPINARDS   mushrooms with spinach and ham stuffing

CHAMPIGNONS FARCIS DE CRABE   mushrooms with crab meat stuffing

CHAMPIGNONS FARCIS DE DUXELLES   mushrooms with minced mushroom stuffing

CHAUD-FROID DE SAUMON   cold salmon in a rich jellied sauce

CHAUSSON   pastry shell stuffed with mussels, fish or meat

CHIFFONNADE DE CRABE   crab, eggs, mayonnaise

COCHONAILLES   sausages and pâtés served as a first course

CORNICHON   small sour pickles or gherkins

CRABE À LA PARISIENNE   crab with mayonnaise and chopped vegetables

CRABE À LA RUSSE   crab in the shell with mayonnaise and capers

CRAQUELOT   smoked, salted herring

CROUSTADE DE CHAMPIGNONS   pastry filled with mushrooms in a sauce

CROUSTADE DE CREVETTES NANTUA   pastry with shrimp in wine sauce

CROUSTADE DE FRUITS DE MER   pastry filled with seafood

CROUSTADE DE MORILLES   morel mushrooms with cream sauce in pastry shell

CROUSTADE JURASSIENNE   pastry shell with bacon and cheese

CROÛTE AUX CHAMPIGNONS   creamed mushrooms in pastry shell

CRUDITÉS   raw salad vegetables

DUCHESSES   pastry shells with various appetizers

ESCARGOTS snails
ESCARGOTS À LA BOURGUIGNONNE snails grilled in garlic butter
ESCARGOTS À LA LANGUEDOCIENNE snails in a spicy sauce
ESCARGOTS À LA NARBONNAISE snails in mayonnaise and ground almonds
ESCARGOTS PETIT-GRIS small land snails
FÈCHE dried pork liver
FILETS D'ANCHOIS fillets of anchovies
FOIE AUX RAISINS chicken liver cooked in wine with grapes
FOIE DE CANARD preserved duck livers
FOIE DE POULET chicken liver
FOIE DE VOLAILLE chicken liver
FOIE GRAS goose liver
FOIE GRAS AUX RAISINS goose liver with grapes
FOIE GRAS EN CROÛTE ground livers baked in pastry
FREMIS lightly cooked oysters
FUMÉE MOULES smoked mussels
GALETTE LAUSANNOISE pastry filled with onions and cheese
GOUGÈRE BOURGUIGNONNE puff pastry shell with Swiss cheese
HARENG FUMÉ smoked herring
HARENG LUCAS smoked herring in mustard mayonnaise sauce
HARENG SALÉ salted kippered herring
HARENG SAUR red herring
HÉNON cockle, like small sea clam
HORS-D'OEUVRE first course
HORS-D'OEUVRE ASSORTIS mixed hors d'oeuvres
HORS-D'OEUVRE RICHE deluxe appetizers
HORS-D'OEUVRE VARIÉS salami and cold meats
JAMBON DE PARME smoked ham eaten raw in paper-thin slices, prosciutto ham
JAMBON FROID cold ham

KIPPER smoked herring
LANGUE À L'ÉCARLATE salted tongue
LIMACE small snail
MAQUEREAU AU VIN BLANC mackerel poached in white wine
MAYONNAISE, CRABE À LA cold crab appetizer
MELON melon
MELON À L'ITALIENNE melon wrapped in thin slices of raw-cured ham
MELON DE CAVAILLON small melon, like canteloupe
MELON GLACÉ iced melon
MELON GLACÉ AU PORTO iced melon pieces in port wine
MELON SUCRIN honeydew melon
MELON SURPRISE melon filled with fruit and liqueur
MOULE mussel
MOULES À LA POULETTE mussels in white sauce with mushrooms
MOULES D'ESPAGNE large raw mussels
MOULES FARCIES stuffed mussels
MOULES MARINIÈRE boiled mussels in white wine with shallots and parsley
MOUSSE DE FOIE GRAS ground goose livers with cream and whipped with truffles
NIÇOISE SALADE salad of vegetables, onions, anchovies, tunafish, artichokes and beans
OEUF DE POISSON egg with fish roe
OEUF SUR CANAPÉ egg, ham and cheese on bread
PÂTÉ minced meat molded, spiced, baked in pastry, served in slices hot or cold
PÂTÉ ARDENNAIS pork and seasonings in pastry
PÂTÉ CHAUD small hot patty filled with meat, fish or grated cheese
PÂTÉ D'AMANDES almond paste
PÂTÉ D'ANGUILLE eel pâté
PÂTÉ DE BÉCASSE woodcock pâté
PÂTÉ D'OIE goose pâté

PÂTÉ DE CAMPAGNE   pork pâté
PÂTÉ DE CANARD   duck pâté
PÂTÉ DE CHEVREUIL   venison pâté
PÂTÉ DE FOIE   liver pâté
PÂTÉ DE FOIE DE PORC   finely ground pork livers
PÂTÉ DE FOIE DE VOLAILLE   chicken liver pâté
PÂTÉ DE FOIE GRAS   goose liver pâté
PÂTÉ DE GIBIER   pâté made with game
PÂTÉ DE GRIVE   pâté made with thrush or songbird
PÂTÉ DE LAPIN   rabbit pâté
PÂTÉ DE LIÈVRE   pâté of wild hare
PÂTÉ DE TÊTE   pâté made from calf's head
PÂTÉ EN CROÛTE   mixture covered with pastry
PÂTÉ FEUILLETÉE   puff pastry
PÂTÉ MAISON   house specialty pâté
PETIT GRATIN DE CRABE AU VIN BLANC   crab meat
   in white wine sauce baked with cheese
PETIT PÂTÉ   small pastry filled with ground meat
PETIT PÂTÉ CHAUD   small hot patty filled with meat or
   fish or grated cheese
PETITE CAISSE DE FROMAGE   cheese and artichoke
   appetizers
PETITES BOUCHÉES   small pastry shells filled with fish
   or other ingredients
PETITS OIGNONS AUX RAISINS   button onions with
   raisins
PILCHARD   sardine
POIREAU À LA NIÇOISE   leek stewed with oil and
   tomatoes
RILLETTE   soft, spreadable pork or goose paste
RILLETTE DE LAPIN   made of pork and rabbit
RILLETTES DE PORC   soft potted pork
ROLLMOPS   pickled herring around a piece of onion
SALADE DE MOULES À LA PROVENÇALE   mussel
   salad with chopped onion fried in olive oil with tom-
   atoes and garlic
SALADE DE QUEUES D'ÉCREVISSES   crayfish salad

SARDINE À L'HUILE   sardine in olive oil

SARDINE NIÇOISE   boneless sardine cooked in white wine, mushrooms and spices

SARDINES AUX OEUFS AU CITRON   sardines with hard boiled eggs and lemon

SAUMON D'ÉCOSSE   Scottish salmon

SAUMON DE NORVÈGE   cold salmon slices in aspic

SAUMON FUMÉ   smoked salmon

SAUMON GLACÉ   cold salmon in aspic jelly

SAUMON PATRICIENNE   salmon on toast with glazed sauce

SAUMON ROSE À LA PARISIENNE   cold poached salmon on mayonnaise and vegetables

TAPENADE   black olives, anchovies, capers, olive oil, lemon juice and tuna fish

TERRINE D'OIE   finely ground goosemeat, usually served as an appetizer

TERRINE DE BROCHET   finely ground pike, usually served as an appetizer

TERRINE MAISON   mixture of chicken, goose livers or pork

TOMATE AU THON À LA MAYONNAISE   tomato stuffed with tuna and mayonnaise

TOMATE FARCIE   stuffed tomato

TOURTELETTE   individual filled pastry

TRUFFE EN CROÛTE   truffle and goose liver in pastry

Beverages

BABEURRE   buttermilk

BIÈRE   beer

CACAO   cocoa

CAFÉ   coffee

CAFÉ ALLONGÉ   weak espresso

CAFÉ AU LAIT   espresso with warmed or lightly steamed milk

CAFÉ CRÈME   espresso with warmed or lightly steamed milk

CAFÉ DÉCAFÉINÉ   decaffeinated coffee
CAFÉ EN POUDRE   instant powder coffee
CAFÉ EXPRESS   plain black espresso
CAFÉ FILTRE   filtered American style coffee
CAFÉ FRAPPÉ   iced coffee
CAFÉ GRAND   large cup of coffee
CAFÉ LIÉGEOIS   iced coffee with ice cream and whipped
   cream
CAFÉ NATURE   black coffee
CAFÉ NOIR   small black coffee
CAFÉ SANS CAFÉINE   caffeine free coffee
CAFÉ SERRÉ   extra strong espresso
CAFÉ SOLUBLE   instant coffee
CAMOMILLE   camomile tea
CARAFE D'EAU   pitcher of tap water
CHOCOLAT CHAUD   hot chocolate
CHOCOLAT EN POUDRE   cocoa
CIDRE   cider
CITRON PRESSÉ   lemon juice with water and sugar for
   sweetening
CITRONNADE   still lemonade
COCA   Coca-Cola
CRÈME   cream
DÉCAFÉINÉ OR DÉCA   decaffeinated espresso
DEMI-TASSE   small cup of strong coffee
DIABOLO   lemonade
DIABOLO MENTHE   mint syrup and lemonade
DOUBLE EXPRESS   a double cup of espresso
EAU   water
EAU GAZEUSE   sparkling soda water
EAU MINÉRALE   mineral water
EAU NATURELLE   water
EXPRESS   espresso coffee
FAUX CAFÉ   decaffeinated coffee
FRAPPÉ   a drink served very cold or with ice
GINI   bitter lemon
GLAÇON   ice cube

GRAIN DE CAFÉ   coffee bean
GRAND CRÈME   large or double espresso with milk
INFUSION   herb tea
JUS DE CITRON   lemon juice
JUS DE FRUITS   fruit juice
JUS DE POMMES   apple juice
JUS DE TOMATE   tomato juice
LAIT   milk
LAIT BARATTÉ   buttermilk
LAIT DEMI-ÉCRÉMÉ   semi skimmed milk
LAIT ÉCRÉMÉ   skimmed milk
LAIT RIBOT   a yogurt drink
LAIT STÉRILISÉ   long life milk
LIMONADE   fizzy lemonade
MANDARIN   bitter, orange flavored drink
MENTHE   sweet, green mint-flavored syrup
MINÉRALE   mineral water
MOKA   coffee, or coffee flavored dish
ORANGE PRESSÉ   fresh squeezed orange juice served
   with a carafe of water and sugar for sweetening
ORANGEADE   orange flavored water
PAMPLEMOUSSE PRESSÉ   grapefruit juice served with
   water and sugar for sweetening
PERRIER   brand of mineral water
PICON   bitter, orange flavored drink
SCHWEPPES   tonic water
THÉ   tea
THÉ AU CITRON   tea with lemon
THÉ AU LAIT   tea with milk
THÉ NATURE   plain tea
TISANE   herb tea
VERVEINE   herb tea

Bread

AILLADE   bread rubbed with oil and garlic
AZYME   unleavened bread

BAGUETTE   crusty white bread loaf
BAGUETTE ANCIENNE   sourdough loaf
BAGUETTE AU LEVAIN   sourdough loaf
BISCOTTE   rusk biscuit
BISCUIT   biscuit
BISTORTO   brioche baked in ring containing aniseed
BOULE   ball, or round loaf
BRETZEL   pretzel
BRIOCHE   sweet roll
CHAPEAU   small round loaf of bread
CHAPELURE   breadcrumbs
COURONNE   ring shaped loaf of bread
CRAMIQUE   bun with currants or raisins
CROISSANT   crescent shaped roll
CROQUET   crisp almond biscuit
CROÛTONS   cubes of toasted or fried bread
DIABLOTIN   cheese croutons served with soup
FARINE   flour
FER À CHEVAL   horseshoe shaped bread
FICELLE   very thin, crusty loaf of bread
FLÛTE   a thin roll
FOUGASSE   crusty, flat bread made of flour, water, yeast,
    may be filled with anchovies or onions
GOUGELHOPF   yeast bread
KOKEBOTEROM   raisin muffin
LÈCHE   thin slice of bread or meat
LIERWECKE   raisin bun
LONGUET   breadstick
MICHE   round loaf of bread
PAIN   bread
PAIN AUX RAISINS   rye or wheat bread filled with raisins
PAIN AZYME   unleavened bread
PAIN BIS   brown bread
PAIN COMPLET   whole-grain bread
PAIN DE CAMPAGNE   country loaf
PAIN DE FROMENT   wheat bread
PAIN DE MIE   sandwich bread

PAIN DE NOIX AND PAIN DE NOISETTES   rye or wheat bread with walnuts or hazelnuts
PAIN DE SEIGLE   bread made from rye flour and some wheat flour
PAIN DE SON   diet bread containing 20% bran
PAIN FANTAISIE   odd shaped bread
PAIN GRILLÉ   toast
PAIN POLKA   large country loaf bread
PAIN RÔTI   toast
PAIN SANS SEL   salt free bread
PAIN VIENNOIS   baguette shaped white bread
PAN BAGNA   roll with tomatoes, anchovies, onions in oil
PETIT PAIN   roll
RÔTIE   slice of toast
SANDWICH MIXTE   gruyere cheese and ham on a baguette
SEIGLE   rye or rye bread
TARTINE   slice of bread
TOURANGELLE, À LA   fried croutons topped with eggs poached in red wine

Butter

BEURRE   butter
BEURRE À L'ORANGE   orange butter for crepes
BEURRE AU CITRON   lemon butter
BEURRE CHIVRY   herb butter
BEURRE CLARIFIÉ   clarified butter
BEURRE DE CREVETTES   shrimp butter
BEURRE GASCOGNE   garlic butter
BEURRE MAÎTRE D'HÔTEL   lemon butter with chopped parsley
BEURRE MANIÉ   paste of flour and butter
BEURRE NOIR   sauce of browned butter, lemon juice or vinegar
BEURRE NOISETTE   lightly browned butter
BEURRE POUR ESCARGOTS   butter, shallot, garlic, and seasoning

BEURRE RAIFORT   horseradish butter
BEURRE VIERGE   butter sauce with salt, pepper and
   lemon juice
BUERRE DE CACAHOUÈTES   peanut butter
HÔTELIÈRE   with parsley butter

Cakes and Pastry

ABAISSE   rolled pastry
ALLELUIA   little cake
BABA AU RHUM   spongecake with rum syrup
BEIGNET   fritter or doughnut
BEIGNET VIENNOIS   deep-fried pastry filled with cream,
   custard or jam
BERAWECKA   fruit cake
BISCUIT   biscuit
BISCUIT AU BEURRE   butter spongecake
BISCUIT CUILLÈRE   ladyfingers
BISCUIT DE REIMS   small macaroon
BISCUIT DE SAVOIE   spongecake
BISCUIT GLACÉ   cracker or biscuit with icing on top
BISCUIT ROULÉ À L'ORANGE ET AUX AMANDES
   orange and almond spongesheet cake
BONBON   sweet or candy
BONVALET   almond cake with ice cream
BRETON, GÂTEAU   rich cake
BRIOCHE   sweet roll
BROYÉ   cereal cake used for dessert
CACCAVELLI   lemon cheesecake
CAJASSE   sweet rum cake
CAJASSE SARLADAISE   rum flavored pastry
CANISTRELLI   almond and hazelnut cake
CASSE-MUSEAU   small cake
CHAMPIGNY   pastry with apricot filling
CHARGOUÈRE   pastry with plums or prunes
CHARLOTTE RUSSE   cream custard with sponge finger cakes
CHAUDE   plum tart

CHAUDEAU   orange tart
CHAUSSON AUX NOISETTES   nut strudel
CHAUSSON AUX POMMES   apple turnover
CHEMISE, EN   wrapped with pastry
CHOUX   cream puff pastry of flour, butter, water and eggs
CITROUILLE, TARTE À LA   pumpkin pie
CLAFOUTIS AUX CERISES   deep-dish cherry cake
COCONS   liqueur flavored marzipan sweets
CONVERSATION   tart with glazing and almond filling
COPEAU DE CHOCOLAT   chocolate shavings as a cake
   decoration
CORDE   sweet pastry
CORRÉZIENNE, GALETTE   walnut filled pastry
COUKEBOOTRAM   cake with raisins
COUP DE JARNAC   spongecake with jam and cognac
COUQUE   cake
CRAMIQUE   bun with currants or raisins
CRAQUELIN   light pastry filled with apple
CROQUANT   crunchy, also small cake made with sugar
   and flour
CROQUET   crisp almond biscuit
CROUSTADE   pastry filled with prunes and apples
DÉLICE   pastry for desserts
DOUCEURS   sweets or desserts
ÉCLAIR AU CHOCOLAT   cream puff with custard cream
   filling, chocolate frosting
FALCULELLI   cheesecake
FANCHETTE   cake with cream filling and meringue
FARINE   flour
FEUILLANTINE   pastry with sugar
FEUILLE AU LAIT   pastry crust filled with custard
FEUILLETÉ   pastry leaves or shell
FEUILLETÉ AUX FRAISES   Napoleon-like pastry with
   strawberries
FLAGNARDE   fruit-filled cake
FLEURONS   puff pastry garnish
FLOTTANTE, ÎLE   cake with whipped cream and custard

FONDANT   frosting for cakes, candies
FOUACE   sweet cake
FRIANDISES   petits fours or cookies
GALETTE   flat round cake
GALICIEN   sponge cake with cream and apricot jam icing
GANACHE   chocolate whipped cream filling for cake
GÂTEAU   cake made without yeast
GÂTEAU À LA BASQUAISE   pastry filled with custard or
   fruit
GÂTEAU À LA PARISIENNE   meringue covered sponge
   cake with almond cream
GÂTEAU ALCAZAR   almond and apricot cake
GÂTEAU AU CHOCOLAT   chocolate cake
GÂTEAU AU FROMAGE   cheese tart
GÂTEAU AUX MARRONS   chestnut cake
GÂTEAU AUX NOISETTES   walnut cake
GÂTEAU GLACÉ   cake and ice cream in slices
GÂTEAU GRENOBLOIS   walnut cake
GÂTEAU LUCULLUS   chocolate chestnut cake
GAUFRETTE   crisp, sweet wafer
GÉNOISE   butter spongecake
GLACE BISCUIT   ice cream on spongecake with fruit,
   liqueur or sauce
GOUGNETTE   sweet fritter
GOYÈRE   cheese tart
GUILLARET   sweet pastry
JARNAC   sponge cake with jam and cognac
JÉSUITE   flaky pastry with almond paste
KAFFEKRANTZ   raisin cake
KOKEBOTEROM   raisin muffin
KOUGLOF   sweet, round Alsatian yeast cake, with
   almonds and raisins
KOUIGN AMANN   puff pastry cake
KUGELHOPF   brioche cake with almonds and raisins
MACARON   macaroon
MADELEINES   small tea cakes
MANQUÉ   spongecake with crystallized fruit

MARIGNAN   cake with liqueur, apricot jam and meringue
MARLY   rum or kirsch flavored cake with strawberries and cream
MARQUISE AU CHOCOLAT   spongecake filled and covered with chocolate cream
MASSEPAIN   almond paste
MAZARIN   spongecake filled with crystallized fruit
MERVEILLE   small cake cooked in oven or deep fried with brandy or rum
MERVEILLES À LA CHARENTAISE   small cakes with cognac
MIGNARDISE   petit four
MILANAIS   spongecake with liqueur, apricot jam and aniseed icing
MILLE-FEUILLE   Napoleon pastry
MILLIASSON   sweet corn flour pastry
MIRLITON   tart with almond-cream filling
MOKATINE   coffee flavored petit four
NANTAIS   almond biscuit
NAPOLITAIN   almond cake with fruit jam
NELUSKO   petit four with brandied cherries and red currant jam
NOISETTINE NONNETTE   two layers of gingerbread pastry with hazelnut cream
NOUGATINE   vanilla spongecake with praline cream and chocolate icing
PAIN DE ÉPICE   gingerbread or spice cake
PAIN D'GÊNES   almond cake
PALMIER   palm leaf shaped cookie made of sugared puff pastry
PARIS-BREST   cream-puff pastry ring with whipped cream filling
PASTA FROLLA   sweet pastry made with kirsch
PASTIS GÉNOISE   spongecake with brandy flavoring
PASTIS LANDAISE   prune filled pastry
PÂTE BRISÉE   pastry used for pies and tarts
PÂTE À CHOUX   cream puff pastry

PÂTISSERIE   pastry

PÂTISSON   orange flavored pastry

PAVÉ AU CHOCOLAT   spongecake with chocolate butter cream and chocolate icing

PETIT FOUR   little filled cakes with sugar frosting topped with candied flowers, nuts or chocolate

PETIT MILLE-FEUILLE   Napoleon; pastry filled with an almond cream sauce and glazed with a sugary mixture

PETITS GÂTEAUX SECS   cookies

PETS DE NONNE   small fried pastry

PITHIVIERS   puff pastry filled with almond cream and rum

POGNE   brioche cake filled with fruit or jam

POMPETTES   orange flavored sweet pastry

PROFITEROLES   pastry filled with ice cream and topped with chocolate sauce

RABOTE   apple in pastry

RAVIOLES   pastries from goats' cheese

REINE DE SABA   chocolate, rum and almond cake

RICHELIEU   almond pastry with apricot jam and almond cream

SABLÉ   shortbread cookie

SALAMBO   small cake filled with kirsch-cream

SAVARIN   ring cake soaked in rum or kirsch

SAVARIN CHANTILLY   cake with kirsch, jam and whipped cream

ST-HONORÉ   iced pastry puffs around cream filled pastry ring

SUCCÈS AU PRALIN   cake flavored with caramelized almonds and frosted with meringue and butter cream

SUCÉE   petit four containing candied fruit

TALIBUR   apple in pastry

TARTE   tart

TARTE À L'ALSACIENNE   custard fruit tart

TARTE MÉGIN   cream cheese tart

TARTOUILLAT   apple tart

TIMBALE DE FRUITS   pastry with apricot jam and cooked fruits on top
TÔT-FAIT   spongecake with lemon
TOURON   candy of almonds, pistachio and crystallized fruit
TOURTEAU AU FROMAGE   goat's milk cheesecake
TUILE   delicate almond flavored cookie
VOL-AU-VENT   large puff pastry shell

Cheese

AISY CENDRÉ   firm, fruity cheese, covered in ash
BANON   soft mild cheese, nutty taste, from goat or sheep milk
BARBEREY   mild, skimmed milk cheese
BEAUMONT   buttery version of Camembert
BELLETOILE TRIPLE-CRÈME   rich, young cheese
BLEU DE BRESSE   strong, salty, fermented, tangy cheese
BLEU DE SAINTE-FOY   crumbly, blue-veined cheese with a sharp taste
BLEU DE SASSENAGE   soft, blue-veined cheese with sharp taste
BOUCHÉE AU FROMAGE   pastry shell with cheese
BOULETTE D'AVESNES   cheese with strong taste and smell, from cow's milk
BOURSAULT   rich, mild, nutty flavor soft cheese
BOURSIN TRIPLE-CRÈME   dessert cheese
BRESSAN   goat's cheese with a slight goaty smell
BRESSE, BLEU DE   blue-veined cheese from cow's milk
BRIE   soft paste cheese with delicate flavor
BRIE DE MEAUX   soft, mild, fermented cheese
BROCHETTE JURASSIENNE   pieces of cheese wrapped in ham and fried
BROUSSE VÉSUBIE   soft and very mild cheese
CABÉCOU   small round goat cheese
CAMEMBERT   soft paste cheese
CANCOILLOTTE   skimmed milk cheese eaten warm on toast

CANTAL   semi-hard cheese
CAPRICE DES DIEUX   mild double-cream cheese
CENDRE DES RICEYS   skimmed-milk cheese with nutty
    taste
CERVELLE CANUT   cheese with herbs wine, and vinegar
CHAMBARAND, TRAPPISTE   soft, mild and creamy
    cheese
CHAOURCE   soft cheese with delicate, fruity taste
CHAROLAIS   cheese from goat's milk
CHEDDAR   cheese
CHÈVRE   a strong goat milk cheese
CHEVRET   goat's milk cheese with a nutty taste
CITEAUX   soft tangy cheese
CLAQUEBITOU   cheese with the taste of herbs and garlic
COMTÉ   semi-hard cheese
COMTÉ, GRUYÈRE DE   firm sharp tasting cows' milk
    cheese
COULOMMIERS   Brie type cheese, similar to Camembert
CROQUE-MADAME   toasted or fried cheese and chicken
    sandwich
CROQUE-MONSIEUR   toasted or fried cheese and ham
    sandwich
CROTTIN DE CHAVIGNOL   firm goat cheese
CROÛTE AU FROMAGE   melted cheese served over toast
DAUPHIN   spicy cheese with strong smell
DEMI SEL   soft cream cheese
DOUBLE-CRÈME   cream cheese
EMMENTAL FRANÇAIS   soft and fruity cheese
ÉPOISSES   soft cheese with an acid taste
EXPLORATEUR   mild cream cheese
FEUILLE DE DREUX   cheese like Brie wrapped in
    chestnut leaves
FEUILLETÉE AU ROQUEFORT   roquefort cheese in puff
    pastry
FLAMMEKUECHE   tart with bacon, onions, cream cheese
FONDU   melted
FONDU AU MARC   soft, mild cheese

FONTAINEBLEAU   cheese made of milk curds and cream
FOURME DE MONBRISON   firm cheese, column-shaped,
  with a bitter taste
FREMGEYE   fresh cream cheese
FROMAGE   cheese
FROMAGE À LA CRÈME   cream cheese
FROMAGE AU MARC DE RAISIN   sweet, usually in a
  crust of grape jelly
FROMAGE BLANC   cream cheese
FROMAGE DE BREBIS   ewe's milk cheese
FROMAGE DE CHÈVRE   goat cheese
FROMAGE DE MONSIEUR   cream cheese
FROMAGE DE VACHE   cow's milk cheese
FROMAGE FRAIS   fresh curd cheese
FROMAGE LE ROI   cream cheese
FROMAGE MAIGRE   low-fat cheese
FROMAGE POUR TARTINER   cheese spread
GÂTEAU AU FROMAGE   cheese tart
GÉRARDMER   mild cow's milk cheese
GÉROMÉ   spicy cheese with a strong smell
GOUGÈRE PÂTE À CHOU   cheese pastry ring
GOYÈRE   cheese tart
GRATIN LANDAIS   potato, ham and cheese dish
GRIS DE LILLE   soft cheese, very spicy
GRUYÈRE   hard, mild Swiss cheese
GRUYÈRE DE BEAUFORT   salty and fruity cow's milk
  cheese
GRUYÈRE DE COMTÉ   firm sharp tasting cows' milk
  cheese
LIVAROT   soft paste cheese
MAMIROLLE   soft, strong cheese
MAROILLES   strong, semi-hard cheese
MIMOLETTE   tangy, semi-hard cheese similar to Edam
MONT D'OR   soft, mild cheese with a delicate taste
MONT DES CATS, ABBAYE DE   soft, mild cheese
MONTRACHET   goat cheese which is wrapped in
  chestnut leaves

MORBIER   firm cheese with black streak and fruity taste
MUNSTER   soft cheese
PAILLETTES   cheese straws made with puff pastry
PARMESANÉ   prepared with parmesan cheese
PERSILLÉ DES ARAVIS   blue-veined, sharp goat's milk
    cheese
PETIT SUISSE   miniature cheese, resembling cream cheese
PICODON DE VALREAS   goat's milk cheese with a nutty
    taste
PIERRE-QUI-VIRE   tangy cheese with strong smell
PLATEAU DE FROMAGES   cheese platter
POIVRE D'ÂNE   cheese made with herbs
PONT-L'ÉVÊQUE   strong soft cheese
PORT SALUT   fairly mild, semi-hard cheese
RACLETTE   melted cheese with boiled potatoes, pickles
    and pickled onions
RAMEQUIN   melted cheese, like a fondue
RAMEQUIN AU FROMAGE   cheese tarts
RÂPÉ, FROMAGE   grated cheese
RAVIOLES   pastries from goats' cheese
REBLOCHON   semi-hard cheese
RIGOTTE CONDRIEU   soft and mild cheese with a milky
    taste
ROLLOT   soft, cow's milk cheese, tangy taste
ROQUEFORT   blue-veined, moist, salty, tangy cheese of
    ewe's milk
SOUFFLÉ AU FROMAGE OEUFS MOLLETS   cheese
    soufflé with boiled eggs
ST-FLORENTIN   tangy, soft cheese like cream cheese
ST-MARCELLIN   strong, creamy cheese
ST-MARCELLIN, TOMME DE   soft and mild cheese
ST-MAURE   creamy, strong goat cheese
ST-PAULIN   semi-hard cheese
ST-REMY   strong smelling spicy cow's milk cheese
TARTE MÉGIN   cream cheese tart
TARTE MOUGIN   tart with eggs, cream and cream cheese
TOMME   mild soft cheese

TOMME ARLÉSIENNE   soft, sheep's milk cheese, very creamy
TOMME AU MARC DE RAISIN   semi-hard cheese
TOMME DE SAVOIE   very mild, semi-soft cheese
VACHERIN ABONDANCE   runny, mild cheese
VACHERIN DU MONT D'OR   firm, mild flavored cows' milk cheese
VALENÇAY   strong creamy goat cheese
VIEUX PUANT   soft, very spicy cheese

Crepes

AUMONIÈRE   filled thin crepe
BEURRE À L'ORANGE   orange butter for crepes
BLINI   thick pancake eaten with caviar
BLINIS AU CAVIAR   thin buckwheat pancakes filled with caviar
CASTAGNACI   chestnut pancakes
CHANCIAU   thick pancake
CRÊPE   thin pancake
CRÊPE À LA VOLAILLE   chicken pancake
CRÊPE DENTELLE   thin pancake with sweet filling
CRÊPES FARCIES JAMBON   pancakes filled with ham and mushrooms
CRÊPES FLORENTINES   crepes with spinach and mushrooms, baked with cheese sauce
CRÊPES FOURRÉES FLAMBÉES   crepes stuffed with orange and almonds
CRÊPES FOURRÉES GRATINÉES   filled French pancakes
CRÊPES JEANETTE   filled with custard, flamed with brandy
CRÊPES NORMANDES   crepes with baked apple slices and caramel
CRÊPES POMMES DE TERRE   grated potato pancakes
CRÊPES ROULÉES FARCIES   crepes with creamed shellfish, gratinéed in wine and cheese sauce
CRÊPES SUZETTE   hot crepe dessert flamed with orange liqueur

FICELLE NORMANDE   pancake with ham, cheese in a
   cream sauce
FICELLE PICARDE   ham and mushroom pancake
GALOPIN   thick pancake with brown sugar
GRANDE CRÊPE   large pancake
JACQUE   apple pancake
MATAFAN   thick potato pancake
PANNEQUET   pancake
POGNON   griddle cake
SANCIAU   thick pancake
SOCCA   chick-pea pancake

Croquettes and Fritters

AIGRETTE   cheese fritter
BEIGNET   fritter or doughnut
BEIGNET ESCURES   pear fritters fried with cream
BEIGNET SOUFFLÉ   fritter with fish or meat filling
BEUGNON   sweet fritter
BIGNON   sweet fritter
BRIGNE   sweet fritter
BUGNE   sweet fritter
CAILLETTE   pork liver and bacon croquette
CASTAGNOLE   batter fritters
COLOMBINE   deep fried croquette with Parmesan cheese
CROQUETTE   ground meat, fish, fowl or vegetables,
   coated in breadcrumbs and deep fried
CRUCHADE   fritter of corn meal
D'ARTAGNAN   stuffed tomato and potato croquettes
FLAMMES   fritters
FRIVOLE   fritter
GAUFRE   waffle
GOUGNETTE   sweet fritter
KNEPFLE   dumpling
METURE   corn fritter
POMME-DE-TERRE, CROQUETTES DE   mashed
   potatoes, deep-fried in breadcrumbs

POMME-DE-TERRE LORETTE　fried potato croquettes
ROUSSETTE　sweet corn flour fritter made with brandy
SUBRIC　croquette of ground meat or fish fried in butter

Desserts and Fruits

ABRICOT　apricot
AEGLE　hybrid tangerine/grapefruit (ugli fruit)
AGRUMES　citrus fruits
AIRELLE　cranberry
AIRELLE ROUGE　cranberry
ALLELUIA　little cake
AMANDE　almond
ANANAS　pineapple
ANANAS MELBA　pineapple on vanilla ice cream with
　raspberry sauce
ARACHIDE　peanut
AVELINE　filbert nut, hazelnut
AVOCAT　avocado
BABA AU RHUM　spongecake with rum syrup
BAIES　berries
BANANE　banana
BANANES SPLIT AU CHOCOLAT　banana with ice
　cream and chocolate sauce
BAR-LE-DUC　currant jelly
BAVAROIS　cream dessert with flavorings and custard
BAVAROIS À L'ORANGE　orange flavored Bavarian
　cream dessert
BEIGNET ESCURES　pear fritters fried with cream
BEIGNET VIENNOIS　deep-fried pastry filled with cream,
　custard or jam
BELLE-ANGEVINE　pear
BELLE-DIJONNAISE　with blackcurrants
BELLE-GARDE　peach
BELLE-HÉLÈNE, POIRE　poached pear with ice cream
　and hot chocolate sauce
BERAWECKA　fruit cake

BERGAMOTE   fruit related to oranges
BERLINGOT   candy with nuts and fruits inside
BEUGNON   sweet fritter
BIGARREAU   red, firm-fleshed variety of cherry
BIGNON   sweet fritter
BISCUIT AU BEURRE   butter spongecake
BISCUIT CUILLÈRE   ladyfingers
BISCUIT DE REIMS   small macaroon
BISCUIT DE SAVOIE   spongecake
BISCUIT GLACÉ   cracker or biscuit with icing on top
BISCUIT ROULÉ À L'ORANGE ET AUX AMANDES
   orange and almond sponge sheet cake
BOMBE   molded frozen dessert
BOMBE AÏDA   tangerine ice with vanilla and kirsch
BOMBE ALHAMBRA   strawberry and vanilla layered ice
   cream
BOMBE DAME-BLANCHE   vanilla ice cream with
   almond mousse
BOMBE FAVORITE   meringue, apricot cream and rum,
   frozen and served with chestnut puree
BOMBE MÉDICIS   ice cream with pear ice, peach mousse
   and kirsch
BOMBE VÉRONIQUE   pistachio and chocolate ice cream
   with grapes
BON-CHRÉTIEN   cooked pear
BONBON   sweet or candy
BONVALET   almond cake with ice cream
BOUDIN POMMES REINETTE   blood pudding with apples
BOULE-DE-NEIGE   ice cream covered with whipped cream
BOULES DE NEIGE AU CHOCOLAT   snowballs of egg
   whites and chocolate
BOURDALOUE   fruit cooked in a light syrup
BOURDANE   apple dumpling
BOURDELOT   apple baked in pastry
BOURDELOT POIRES   baked pears
BOURSIN TRIPLE-CRÈME   dessert cheese
BRETON, GÂTEAU   rich cake

BRIGNE   sweet fritter
BRIGNOLE   dried plum
BROYÉ   cereal cake used for dessert
BRUGNON   nectarine
BRÛLÉ   burned or caramelized
BUGNE   sweet fritter
CACAHOUÈTES   peanuts
CACCAVELLI   lemon cheesecake
CAFÉ GLACÉ   coffee flavored ice cream dessert
CAFÉ LIÉGEOIS   iced coffee with ice cream and whipped
   cream
CAILLÉ   clotted or curdled
CAJASSE   sweet, rum cake
CAJASSE SARLADAISE   rum flavored pastry
CAJOU, NOUX DE   cashew nut
CALISSON   marzipan sweet
CANISTRELLI   almond and hazelnut cake
CANNEBERGE   cranberry
CAPRICE   a dessert
CARAMEL   cooked confection
CASSATE   ice cream dessert made with fruits
CASSE-MUSEAU   small cake
CASSIS   black currant
CASSISSINE   black currant sweet candy or stuffing
CÉDRAT   sour lemon
CERISE   cherry
CERISE NOIRE   black cherry
CERISES JUBILÉE   cherries flamed in brandy over ice cream
CERNEAU   green walnut meat
CHADEAU   a rich dessert type sauce
CHAMPIGNY   pastry with apricot filling
CHANTILLY   sweetened whipped cream
CHARENTAIS   sweet melon
CHARGOUÈRE   pastry with plums or prunes
CHARIOT À DESSERTS   rolling cart carrying varied desserts
CHARLOTTE   molded dessert with ladyfingers and
   custard filling

CHARLOTTE AUX POMMES molded apple dessert
CHARLOTTE MALAKOFF AU CHOCOLAT chocolate-almond cream molded in ladyfingers
CHARLOTTE RUSSE cream custard with sponge finger cakes
CHÂTAIGNE small chestnut
CHAUDE plum tart
CHAUDEAU orange tart
CHAUSSON AUX NOISETTES nut strudel
CHAUSSON AUX POMMES apple turnover
CHOCOLAT chocolate
CHOCOLAT AMER bittersweet chocolate
CHOCOLAT AU LAIT milk chocolate
CHOUX cream puff pastry of flour, butter, water and eggs
CIGARETTE tubular petit four served with ice cream
CITRON lemon
CITRON VERT lime
CITRONNAT candied lemon peel
CITROUILLET, TARTE À LA pumpkin pie
CLAFOUTIS tart of batter, fruit and black cherries
CLAFOUTIS AUX CERISES deep-dish cherry cake
CLÉMENTINE tangerine
COCO, NOIX DE coconut
COCONS liqueur flavored marzipan sweets
COING quince
COLONEL lemon sherbet doused with vodka
COMPOTE stewed fruit
COMPOTE D'ABRICOTS stewed fresh apricots
COMPOTE DE FRUITS fruit poached in vanilla syrup
CONDÉ rice with fruits
CONFITURE jam
CONFITURE À L'ORANGE marmalade
CONSERVE canned or preserved
CONVERSATION tart with glazing and almond filling
COPEAU DE CHOCOLAT chocolate shavings as a cake decoration
CORBEILLE DE FRUITS basket of fruit

CORDE   sweet pastry
CORNET   slice of ham or tongue rolled and stuffed; also an ice cream cone
CORRÉZIENNE, GALETTE   walnut filled pastry
COUKEBOOTRAM   cake with raisins
COULIS   puree of raw or cooked vegetables or fruit
COUP DE JARNAC   spongecake with jam and cognac
COUPE   dessert with ice cream and fruit
COUPE GLACÉE   sundae
COUPE JACQUES   ice cream with fruit in kirsch liqueur
COUQUE   cake
CRAQUELIN   light pastry filled with apple
CRÈME   cream
CRÈME ANGLAISE   custard sauce
CRÈME ANGLAISE AU CHOCOLAT   soft chocolate custards
CRÈME AU BEURRE À L'ANGLAISE   custard butter cream
CRÈME AU BEURRE AU SIROP   French butter cream made with sugar syrup
CRÈME AU BUERRE À LA MERINGUE   meringue butter cream
CRÈME BRÛLÉE   rich custard dessert with a top of caramelized sugar
CRÈME CARAMEL   caramel custard
CRÈME CHANTILLY   sweetened whipped cream
CRÈME ÉPAISSE   thick cream
CRÈME FOUETTÉE   whipped cream
CRÈME FRAÎCHE   lightly soured cream
CRÈME GLACÉE   ice cream
CRÈME HOMÈRE   egg custard with honey, wine
CRÈME MERINGUÉE   a type of egg custard decorated with fruits
CRÈME MOULE   baked custard dessert
CRÈME PÂTISSIÈRE   custard cream filling
CRÈME PLOMBIÈRES   custard filled with fresh fruits and egg whites

CRÈME RENVERSÉE   vanilla custard or flan
CRÈME SABAYON   an egg yolk and wine dessert
CRÊPES FOURRÉES FLAMBÉES   crepes stuffed with
   orange and almonds
CRÊPES JEANETTE   filled with custard, flamed with brandy
CRÊPES NORMANDES   crepes with baked apple slices
   and caramel
CRÊPES SUZETTE   hot crepe dessert flamed with orange
   liqueur
CROQUEMBOUCHE   crisp profiteroles filled with cream
   and sugar glaze
CROUSTADE   pastry filled with prunes and apples
DAME BLANCHE   peaches in syrup with vanilla ice cream
   and pineapple, in kirsch, with whipped cream
DATTE   date
DÉLICE   pastry for desserts
DIPLOMATE   custard dessert with candied fruit and lady
   fingers
DOUCEURS   sweets or desserts
DOUILLON   pear baked in pastry
DRAGÉE   sugar-coated almond or sweet
ÉCLAIR AU CHOCOLAT   cream puff with custard cream
   filling, chocolate frosting
ENTREMETS   sweets
FAINE   beechnut
FALCULELLI   cheesecake
FANCHETTE   cake with cream filling and meringue
FANTAISIE BOURBONNAISE   baked apricot dessert
FAR BRETON   sweet pudding with prunes
FARCE DE FRAISES CIO-CIO-SAN   strawberry filling
   with almonds and kumquats
FEUILLANTINE   pastry with sugar
FEUILLE AU LAIT   pastry crust filled with custard
FEUILLETÉ AUX FRAISES   Napoleon like pastry with
   strawberries
FIGUE   fig
FIGUE DE BARBARIE   prickly pear

FLAGNARDE   fruit-filled cake

FLAN   sweet or savory custard

FLANGNARDE   sweet vanilla pudding baked in a dish

FLOTTANTE, ÎLE   cake with whipped cream and custard

FONDANT   frosting for cakes, candies

FOUACE   sweet cake

FOUETTÉE   whipped

FRAISE   strawberry

FRAISES DES BOIS   small wild strawberries

FRAISES MARGUERITE   strawberries with kirsch, sherbet and whipped cream

FRAISES MELBA   strawberries with vanilla ice cream, sauce of strawberries or raspberries

FRAISES ROMANOFF   strawberries in orange flavored liqueur and whipped cream

FRAMBOISE   raspberry, also raspberry liqueur

FRANGIPANE   almond custard filling

FRIANDISES   petits fours or cookies

FRUIT   fruit

FRUIT CONFIT   candied fruit or preserved fruit

FRUIT DE LA PASSION   passion fruit

FRUITS CUITS   stewed fruit

FRUITS FRAIS   fresh fruit

FRUITS RAFRAÎCHIS   fruit salad

GALABART   black pudding

GALICIEN   spongecake with cream and apricot jam icing

GANACHE   chocolate whipped cream filling for cake

GÂTEAU   cake made without yeast

GÂTEAU À LA BASQUAISE   pastry filled with custard or fruit

GÂTEAU À LA PARISIENNE   meringue covered spongecake with almond cream

GÂTEAU ALCAZAR   almond and apricot cake

GÂTEAU AU CHOCOLAT   chocolate cake

GÂTEAU AUX MARRONS   chestnut cake

GÂTEAU AUX NOISETTES   walnut cake

GÂTEAU GLACÉ   cake and ice cream in slices

GÂTEAU GRENOBLOIS   walnut cake

GÂTEAU LUCULLUS   chocolate chestnut cake

GAUFRETTE   crisp, sweet wafer

GELÉE DE GROSEILLES   currant jelly

GENIÈVRE   juniper berry

GÉNOISE   butter spongecake

GIVRÉ, FRUIT   citrus fruit sorbets

GLACE   ice cream

GLACE À LA VANILLE   vanilla ice cream

GLACE AUX FRAISES   strawberry ice cream

GLACE BISCUIT   ice cream on spongecake with fruit,
     liqueur or sauce

GLACE NAPOLITAINE   ice cream of different flavors

GOYÈRE   cheese tart

GRAIN DE RAISIN   grape

GRAMOLATE   sherbet

GRENADE   pomegranate

GRIOTTES   red, sour cherries

GROSEILLE   currant

GROSEILLE À MAQUEREAU   gooseberry

GROSEILLE BLANCHE   white currant

GROSEILLE ROUGE   red currant

GUIGNE   cherry

GUILLARET   sweet pastry

ÎLE FLOTTANTE   spongecake sprinkled with kirsch,
     maraschinos, currants, almonds and covered with crème
     anglaise

IMPÉRATRICE (RIZ À L')   rice pudding dessert with
     candied fruit

JARNAC   spongecake with jam and cognac

JÉSUITE   flaky pastry with almond paste

KAFFEKRANTZ   raisin cake

KAKI   persimmon

KISSEL   dessert of mixed berries with cream cheese

KOUGLOF   sweet, round Alsatian yeast cake, with
     almonds and raisins

KOUIGN AMANN   puff pastry cake

KUGELHOPF   brioche cake with almonds and raisins
KUMQUAT   miniature orange
LIÉGEOIS   soft ice cream dessert
LIMON   lime
MACARON   macaroon
MACÉDOINE DE FRUITS   diced mixed fruit or vegetables
MADELEINES   small tea cakes
MANDARINE   tangerine
MANGUÉ   mango
MANQUE   spongecake with crystallized fruit
MARIGNAN   cake with liqueur, apricot jam and meringue
MARLY   rum or kirsch flavored cake with strawberries
    and cream
MARQUISE AU CHOCOLAT   spongecake filled and
    covered with chocolate cream
MARRON   large chestnut
MARRON GLACÉ   candied chestnut
MASSEPAIN   almond paste
MAZARIN   spongecake filled with crystallized fruit
MELON   melon
MELON D'EAU   watermelon
MELON DE CAVAILLON   small melon, like canteloupe
MELON FRAPPÉ   melon filled with sherbet
MELON GLACÉ   iced melon
MELON GLACÉ AU PORTO   iced melon pieces in port wine
MELON SUCRIN   honeydew melon
MELON SURPRISE   melon filled with fruit and liqueur
MERINGUE   stiffly beaten egg whites
MERINGUE AUX NOISETTES   meringue with toasted nuts
MERINGUE GLACÉE   beaten egg whites baked and
    cooled, and served with ice cream
MERINGUE ITALIENNE   sugar-syrup meringue mixture
MERINGUETTES   baked finger lengths of stiffly beaten
    egg whites
MERVEILLE   small cake cooked in oven or deep fried
    with brandy or rum
MERVEILLES À LA CHARENTAISE   small cakes with cognac

MIEL   honey

MIGNARDISE   petit four

MILANAIS   spongecake with liqueur, apricot jam and aniseed icing

MILLASSOU   sweet corn custard

MILLE-FEUILLE   Napoleon pastry

MILLIASSON   sweet corn flour pastry

MIRABELLES   small yellow-green plums

MIRLITONS   tart with almond-cream filling

MOKATINE   coffee flavored petit four

MONT BLANC   dessert of mashed chestnuts and whipped cream

MONTÉ-CRISTO   flan with almond filling

MOUSSE   beaten egg whites or whipped cream; meat, poultry or fish finely ground and served in a mold

MOUSSE AU CHOCOLAT   chocolate, egg yolks, sugar, beaten to mousse consistency

MOUSSE GLACÉE AUX FRAISES   strawberry sherbet whipped until frothy

MÛRE   blackberry

MÛRE SAUVAGE   wild blackberry

MUSCADELLE   pear

MYRTILLE   blueberrylike berry

MYSTÈRE   dessert of meringue, ice cream and chocolate sauce

NAPOLITAIN   almond cake with fruit jam

NAPOLITAINE   vanilla, strawberry and chocolate ice cream, sliced

NÈGRE EN CHEMISE   chocolate dessert with whipped cream

NEIGE, CITRON À LA   lemon flavored shaved ice

NELUSKO   petit four with brandied cherries and red currant jam

NESSELRODE   dessert or sauce containing fruits, chestnuts and whipped cream

NOISETTE   hazelnut, also small round piece, as of potato, generally size of a hazelnut, lightly browned in butter

NOISETTINE NONNETTE   two layers of gingerbread pastry with hazelnut cream

NOIX   nuts in general, but also walnuts

NOIX DE BRÉSIL   Brazil nuts

NOIX DE COCO   coconut

NORMANDE, À LA   fish or meat cooked with apple cider; apple dessert with cream

NOUGAT   sweet candy made of almonds and nougat

NOUGAT GLACÉ   burnt almond ice cream

NOUGATINE   vanilla spongecake with praline cream and chocolate icing

OEUF À LA NEIGE   egg white sweetened and poached in milk and vanilla custard

OLIVES FARCIES NOIRES   stuffed black olives

OLIVES FARCIES VERTES   stuffed green olives

OLIVES NOIRES   black olives

OLIVES VERTES   green olives

OMELETTE FLAMBÉE AU RHUM   dessert omelet with flaming rum

OMELETTE NORVÉGIENNE   ice cream with meringue topping baked, like Baked Alaska

OMELETTE SOUFFLÉE À LA LIQUEUR   liqueur flavored souffle

OMELETTE SURPRISE   meringue and ice cream, browned on top, like Baked Alaska

ORANGE   orange

ORANGE GIVRÉE   orange ice or sherbet in an orange shell

PAIN D'ÉPICE   gingerbread or spice cake

PAIN DE GÊNES   almond cake

PALISSADE DE MARRONS   molded chestnut and chocolate dessert

PALMIER   palm leaf shaped cookie made of sugared puff pastry

PAMPLEMOUSSE   grapefruit

PAPAYE   papaya fruit

PARFAIT   a dessert of ice cream, whipped cream and fruits

PARFUMS DIVERS   different flavors

PARIS-BREST   cream-puff pastry ring with whipped cream filling

PASTA FROLLA   sweet pastry made with kirsch

PASTÈQUE   watermelon

PASTILLE   hard candy of flavored sugar

PASTIS GÉNOISE   spongecake with brandy flavoring

PASTIS LANDAISE   prune filled pastry

PÂTE À CHOUX   cream puff pastry

PÂTISSON   orange flavored pastry

PAVÉ AU CHOCOLAT   spongecake with chocolate butter cream and chocolate icing

PÊCHE   peach

PÊCHE ALEXANDRA   poached peach with ice cream and pureed berries

PÊCHE CARDINAL   poached peaches with raspberry puree

PÊCHE MELBA   vanilla ice cream with peaches in raspberry puree

PETIT FOUR   little filled cakes with sugar frosting topped with candied flowers, nuts or chocolate

PETIT MILLE-FEUILLE   Napoleon; pastry filled with an almond cream sauce and glazed with a sugary mixture

PETIT POT DE CRÈME   little pot of cream, cold custard

PETIT POT DE CRÈME À LA VANILLE   small vanilla custard

PETIT POT DE CRÈME AU CHOCOLAT   chocolate cream custard

PETITS GÂTEAUX SECS   cookies

PIGNON   pine nut

PISTACHE   pistachio nut

PITHIVIERS   puff pastry filled with almond cream and rum

PLOMBIÈRES   dessert of vanilla ice cream, candied fruit, kirsch, and sweetened whipped cream

POGNE   brioche cake filled with fruit or jam

POIRE   pear

POIRE ALMA   pear poached in wine

POIRE AU GRATIN   pear baked with wine and macaroons

POIRE BELLE HÉLÈNE   pear with vanilla ice cream and
   chocolate sauce
POIRE CARDINAL   cooked pears with raspberry sauce
   and toasted almonds
POIRE CONDÉ   hot pear on vanilla flavored rice
POIRE POCHÉE AU VIN ROUGE   pear poached in red wine
POMME   apple
POMME BELLE VUE   molded apple custard
POMME BONNE FEMME   baked apple
POMME EN L'AIR   caramelized apple slices
POMME SAUVAGE   wild crabapple
POMPETTES   orange flavored sweet pastry
POT-DE-CRÈME   individual custard dessert
POUDING   pudding
PRALIN   brittle of almonds, walnuts, hazelnuts, pecans
   and caramel
PRALIN DE NOIX   caramelized walnut brittle
PROFITEROLES   pastry filled with ice cream and topped
   with chocolate sauce
PRUNE   plum
PRUNEAUX   dried prunes
PUITS D'AMOUR   pastry shell with liqueur flavored custard
PURÉE DE POMMES   applesauce
QUETSCH   small purple plum
RABOTE   apple in pastry
RAFRAÎCHIS FRUITS   chilled fruit salad
RAISIN   grape
RAISIN DE CORINTHE   raisin
RAISINÉ   grape jelly
RÉGLISSE   liquorice
REINE CLAUDE   plum
REINE DE SABA   chocolate, rum and almond cake
RICHELIEU   almond pastry with apricot jam and almond
   cream
RIZ AU LAIT   rice custard
RIZ IMPÉRATRICE   Bavarian cream with rice, fruits and kirsch

SABLÉ   shortbread cookie
SALAMBO   small cake filled with kirsch-cream
SAVARIN   ring cake soaked in rum or kirsch
SAVARIN CHANTILLY   cake with kirsch, jam and
  whipped cream
SIROP   syrup
SORBET   sherbet made with water
SOUFFLÉ   light, sweet or piquant mixture served either
  hot or cold, containing whipped egg whites to puff up
  when baked
SOUFFLÉ À L'ORANGE, FLAMBÉ   rum, orange and
  macaroon soufflé, flamed
SOUFFLÉ AU CHOCOLAT   chocolate soufflé
SOUFFLÉ AUX FRAMBOISES   raspberry soufflé
SOUFFLÉ AUX FRUITS   soufflé made with fruit preserves
  or pieces of fruit
SOUFFLÉ GRAND MARNIER   orange liqueur soufflé
SOUFFLÉ PALMYRE   soufflé made with macaroons or
  cake crumbs
SOUFFLÉ ROTHSCHILD   vanilla souffle with fruit
SPUMONI   mixed flavored ice cream with candied fruit
ST-HONORÉ   iced pastry puffs around cream filled pastry ring
SUCCÈS AU PRALIN   cake flavored with caramelized
  almonds and frosted with meringue and butter cream
SUCÉE   petit-four containing candied fruit
SUSPENS   ice cream covered with chopped nuts
TALIBUR   apple in pastry
TARTE   tart
TARTE À L'ALSACIENNE   custard fruit tart
TARTE AUX FRAISES   fresh strawberry flan
TARTE AUX FRUITS   fruit tart
TARTE AUX POMMES   apple tart
TARTE MAISON   tart prepared in the manner of the
  restaurant
TARTE TATIN   caramelized upside down apple pie,
  served warm

TARTELETTES   little tarts filled with various ingredients
TARTOUILLAT   apple tart
TEMPLE GLACÉ À LA MARTINIQUAISE   mold of ice cream with rum and chocolate
TIMBALE DE FRUITS   pastry with apricot jam and cooked fruits on top
TÔT-FAIT   spongecake with lemon
TOURON   candy of almonds, pistachio and crystallized fruit
TOURTEAU AU FROMAGE   goat's milk cheesecake
TRANCHE NAPOLITAINE   ice cream and crystallized fruit
TRIPOTCHA   spicy pudding
TUILE   delicate almond flavored cookie
VACHERIN   meringue case for dessert creams, ice creams or fruit and berry mixtures
VACHERIN GLACÉ   ice cream dessert with meringue
VALENCE, ORANGE DE   Valencia orange
VALLÉE D'AUGE   garnish of cooked apples and cream
VANILLE   vanilla
VARIÉ   assorted or varied
VIN, ORANGE AU   orange sections in white wine
WILLIAM   sweet pear
YAOURT   yogurt
YAOURT À LA CONFITURE   with preserves
ZESTE   peel of orange or lemon

Eggs

AURORE, OEUF À L'   stuffed egg, grated cheese, with tomato sauce
AÎOLI   garlicky blend of eggs and olive oil
DIABLE, OEUF À LA   fried egg with vinegar
DORÉ   browned, with egg yolk
JAUNE D'OEUF   egg yolk
MAYONNAISE   dressing of egg yolks, vinegar or lemon juice
MIMOSA   garnish of chopped, hard-boiled egg yolks
OEUF   egg, also see omelettes

OEUF À L'AGENAISE   baked egg with fried eggplant and onion

OEUF À L'AUTRICHIENNE   poached egg with cabbage and sausages

OEUF À L'HONGROISE   hard egg with onions and mayonnaise

OEUF À LA BRETONNE   egg stuffed with onions, mushrooms and leeks

OEUF À LA DIABLE   deviled egg

OEUF À LA FLORENTINE   egg served with spinach

OEUF À LA LORRAINE   egg baked with cheese and bacon

OEUF À LA MAZARINE   egg custard with tomato sauce

OEUF À LA MÉNAGÈRE   fried egg on macaroni with tomato sauce

OEUF À LA PARISIENNE   baked egg, mushrooms and ground chicken

OEUF À LA PÉRIGOURDINE   egg baked with ground goose liver

OEUF À LA RUSSE   hard egg yolk mixed with mayonnaise and herbs

OEUF AMIRAL   egg mixed with pieces of lobster

OEUF ARGENTEUIL   scrambled egg with asparagus tips

OEUF AU BEURRE NOIR   egg with brown butter

OEUF AU JAMBON   ham and egg

OEUF AU LARD   egg with bacon

OEUF AUX AUBERGINES FRITES   egg with fried eggplant

OEUF BELLEVILLOISE   baked egg in a cream sauce with sausage

OEUF BÉNÉDICTINE   poached egg with ham and hollandaise sauce

OEUF BERCY   baked egg with sausage and tomato sauce

OEUF BROUILLÉ   scrambled egg

OEUF CHASSEUR   scrambled egg with chicken livers

OEUF COCOTTE   egg baked in custard cups with cream

OEUF COCOTTE À LA REINE AUX TOMATES   baked egg with macaroni, tomatoes and Béchamel sauce

OEUF COQUE   boiled egg

OEUF DE POISSON   egg with fish roe
OEUF DUR   hard-boiled egg
OEUF DUR À LA TRIPE   hard-boiled egg in onion sauce
OEUF EN GELÉE   poached egg in aspic or wine flavored jelly
OEUF EN MEURETTE   poached egg in red wine sauce
OEUF FARCIS   stuffed eggs
OEUF FRITS   fried egg
OEUF GRAND-DUC   poached egg in mornay sauce with asparagus tips
OEUF LUCULLUS   poached egg on artichoke heart in cream sauce with foie gras
OEUF MIRETTE   tart with a poached egg yolk and chicken in a cream sauce
OEUF MOLLET   five-minute boiled egg
OEUF PASCAL   egg baked in mustard and cream sauce
OEUF POCHÉ   poached egg
OEUF POCHÉ EN MEURETTE   poached egg in red wine sauce
OEUF POCHÉ SOUFFLÉ À LA FLORENTINE   soufflé of poached egg on creamed spinach
OEUF POÊLÉ   sunny-side-up fried egg
OEUF ROSSINI   egg, truffles and Madeira wine
OEUF SUR CANAPÉ   egg, ham and cheese on bread
OEUFS À L'AGENAISE   baked eggs with fried eggplant and onion
OMELETTE   eggs usually whipped with other ingredients, also see oeufs
OMELETTE À L'ALGÉRIENNE   omelette with eggplant and artichokes
OMELETTE À L'ESPAGNOLE   omelette with tomato sauce, onions, Spanish omelette
OMELETTE À L'OIGNONS   omelette with sautéed onions
OMELETTE À LA BASQUAISE   omelette with green peppers, tomatoes and ham
OMELETTE AU CHOIX   omelette with filling of your choice
OMELETTE AU FOIE DE VOLAILLE   omelette with chicken liver

OMELETTE AU FROMAGE   omelette with cheese

OMELETTE AU FROMAGE AU JAMBON   omelette with cheese or ham

OMELETTE AU GRUYÈRE   omelette with Swiss Cheese

OMELETTE AUX CROUTONS   omelette with fried bread

OMELETTE AUX ÉPINARDS   omelette with spinach

OMELETTE AUX FINES HERBES   omelette with herbs

OMELETTE AUX FRUITS DE MER   omelette with seafood

OMELETTE AUX POINTES D'ASPERGES   omelette with asparagus

OMELETTE AUX TOMATES   omelette with tomato

OMELETTE AUX TRUFFES   omelette with truffles

OMELETTE BONNE FEMME   omelette with onions and chopped bacon

OMELETTE CÉLESTINE   omelette with mushrooms

OMELETTE CLAMART   omelette with fresh peas and green onions

OMELETTE DE CREVETTES   omelette with shrimp

OMELETTE FLAMBÉE AU RHUM   dessert omelette with flaming rum

OMELETTE GRATINÉE AUX CHAMPIGNONS   omelette with mushroom and cheese sauce

OMELETTE LIMOUSINE   omelette with fried potatoes and ham

OMELETTE LYONNAISE   omelette with onions

OMELETTE MAINTENON   omelette with chicken and mushrooms in white onion sauce with browned cheese

OMELETTE NATURE   whipped eggs, pancake style

OMELETTE NIÇOISE   omelette with tomato and anchovies

OMELETTE NORMANDE   omelette with mushrooms and shrimps

OMELETTE PARISIENNE   omelette with onion, mushroom and sausages

OMELETTE PARMENTIER   omelet with boiled potatoes

OMELETTE PROVENÇALE   omelette with garlic, tomatoes and onions

OMELETTE SAVOYARDE   omelette with leeks, potatoes and cheese

OMELETTE SOUFFLÉ À LA LIQUEUR   liqueur flavored soufflé

PIPERADE   scrambled eggs, pepper, onions, tomatoes and ham

POCHÉ   poached egg

QUICHE LORRAINE   egg and cheese pie

SOUFFLÉ AU FROMAGE OEUFS MOLLETS   cheese soufflé with boiled eggs

SOUFFLÉE, OMELETTE   puffy omelet

TARTE MOUGIN   tart with eggs, cream and cream cheese

TOURANGELLE, À LA   fried croutons topped with eggs poached in red wine

Fondues

FONDUE BOURGUIGNONNE   pieces of meat dipped into boiling oil and eaten with various sauces

FONDUE CHINOISE   thin slices of beef dipped into boiling bouillon then eaten with various sauces

FONDUE DE FROMAGE   melted cheese, wine, kirsch into which bread is dipped

FONDUE FORESTIÈRE   sautéed with mushrooms, potatoes and bacon

Game

AILE   wing of poultry or game bird

AILERON   wing tip

ALOUETTE   lark; also a lamb dish made with shoulder, curry and cream

AVOCETTE   pigeon size bird similar to a wild duck

BARAQUILLE   triangular pastry filled with game

BÉCASSE   woodcock

BÉCASSINE   snipe

BECFIGUE   bird usually grilled on a skewer
BICHE   female deer
CAILLE   quail
CANARD À L'ORANGE   roast duck braised with oranges
    and orange liqueur
CANARD AUX CERISES   duck with cherries
CANARD AUX OLIVES   duck cooked with olives
CANARD NANTAIS   delicate flavored small duck
CANARD ROUEN   cross between domestic and wild duck
CANARD SAUVAGE   wild duck
CANETON   duckling
CANETON À L'ORANGE   duckling with orange
CANETON À LA BIGARADE   duckling with bitter oranges
CANETON AUX CERISES   duckling with cherries
CANETON AUX NAVETS   duck with turnips
CANETON AUX OLIVES   duck with olives
CANETON MONTMORENCY   roast duck with poached
    cherries in a port sauce
CERF   venison
CHAMOIS   wild antelope
CHASSEUR, CONSOMMÉ   game consommé, madeira
    and mushrooms
CHEVREUIL   young roe deer
CIMIER   venison hip
CIVET   stew of game thickened with blood
CIVET DE LAPIN   rabbit stewed in wine
CIVET DE LIÈVRE   hare stewed in wine
CIVET DE LIÈVRE À LA FRANCAISE   hare cooked in
    wine, mushrooms and onions
COLOMBE   dove
COLVERT   wild duck
CONFIT D'OIE   goose preserved in its own fat in earthen jars
CONFIT DE CANARD   pieces of duck cooked and pre-
    served in earthen jars
COQ DE BRUYÈRE   grouse
CORBEAU   crow
CÔTELETTES DE CHEVREUIL   venison cutlets

CUISSOT   hip of venison
DODINE DE CANARD   duck stewed with onions
FAISAN   pheasant
FAISAN À LA CRÈME   pheasant in cream sauce
FAISAN NORMAND   casserole of pheasant with salt
   pork, butter, apples, sour cream, pepper, applejack
FAISAN VALLÉE D'AUGE   pheasant with apples and cream
FAISANDÉ   aged game
FOIE DE CANARD   preserved duck livers
FOIE GRAS AUX RAISINS   goose liver with grapes
FOIE GRAS EN CROÛTE   ground livers baked in pastry
GARENNE, LAPIN DE   wild rabbit
GELINOTTE   prairie chicken or grouse
GIBELOTTE   fricassee of rabbit in wine
GIBELOTTE DE LAPIN   rabbit stew with wine sauce
GIBIER   game
GIBIER À PLUME   feathered game
GIBIER À POIL   furred game
GIBIER DE SAISON   game in season
GIGUE   haunch or hip of game meats
GRIVE   thrush
HÉRISSON   hedgehog
HIRONDELLE   swallow
HUITRIER   marsh bird
LANGUEDOCIENNE, PÂTÉ DE PIGEON À LA   pigeon
   pie with mushrooms and chicken livers
LAPEREAU   young rabbit
LAPIN   rabbit
LAPIN À LA HAVRAISE   roast rabbit with bacon in
   cream sauce
LAPIN DE GARENNE   wild rabbit
LIÈVRE   hare
LIÈVRE À LA PIRON   hare marinated and roasted in a
   peppery cream sauce
LIÈVRE À LA ROYALE   dish of hare, ground livers, wine
   and truffles
MAGRET DE CANARD   breast of duck, grilled rare

MARCASSIN   young wild boar

MARCASSIN À L'ARDENNAISE   roasted wild boar in red wine sauce

MARCASSIN FARCI AU SAUCISSON   boar stuffed with sausage

MAUVIETTE   wild meadowlark or skylark game birds

OISEAU   bird

ORTOLAN   small game bird like a finch

PALOMBE   wood or wild pigeon

PÂTÉ CHARTRES   partridge in pastry

PERDRIX   partridge

PERDRIX À LA CATALANE   partridge stew

PERDRIX À LA VIGNERONNE   partridges with grapes

PERDRIX AUX CHOUX   casseroled partridge with cabbage

PIGEON À LA RUSSE   squab or pigeon cooked with a sour cream sauce

PIGEONNEAU   squab

PIGEONNEAU AUX POIS   baked squab with peas, onions, pork, chicken broth

PIGEONNEAU SUR CANAPÉ   roast squab on liver canape

PINTADE   guinea fowl

PINTADE AUX LENTILLES   guinea hen with lentils

PINTADE FORESTIÈRE   guinea hen with pork, onions, potatoes, broth, mushrooms

PINTADEAU   young guinea fowl

PINTADEAU AUX GIROLLES   guinea fowl stuffed with mushrooms, braised in wine

PINTADEAU EN COCOTTE   guinea fowl braised in a casserole

PINTADEAU MONSOLET   guinea fowl stuffed with goose liver, braised with artichokes

PINTADEAU RICHELIEU   guinea fowl fried in butter with lemon juice

PINTADEAU SALMI   guinea fowl braised with onions, mushrooms, Madeira wine

PINTADEAU SOUVAROFF   guinea fowl stuffed with goose liver, braised in Madeira wine

POULE FAISANE   female pheasant

RÂBLE DE LIÈVRE   saddle of rabbit

SALMIS   stewlike preparation of game birds or poultry in wine

SALMIS DE PALOMBES   roast pigeon, wine, onions, ham and mushrooms

SANGLIER   wild boar

SANGLIER, CUISSOT DE   haunch of wild boar

SANGLIER, SELLE DE   saddle of wild boar

SARCELLE   teal, small duck

SAUTÉ DE LAPIN AU VIN BLANC   rabbit stewed in white wine sauce

TERRINE   earthenware container for baking meat, game, fish or vegetable mixture

TERRINE DE CAILLE   quail cooked in an earthenware container

TERRINE DE CANARD   duck cooked in an earthenware container

TERRINE DE FAISAN   pheasant cooked in an earthenware container

TERRINE DE GIBIER   wild game pâté

TERRINE DE GRIVES   thrush cooked in an earthenware container

TERRINE DE LAPIN   rabbit pâté

TERRINE DE PERDREAU   partridge cooked in an earthenware container

TÉTRAS   grouse

TOURTE DE CANETON   duck baked in a pie

VENAISON   venison

Grains and Cereals

AVOINE   oats

AVOINE, FARINE D'   oatmeal

BLÉ   wheat

CÉRÉALE   cereal

FAR   porridge

FARINE COMPLÈTE   wholewheat flour
FARINE D'AVOINE   oat flour
FARINE DE BLÉ   wheat flour
FARINE DE SARRASIN   buckwheat flour
FARINE DE SEIGLE   rye flour
FLOCONS DE MAÎS   corn flakes
GAUDES   corn flour porridge
GRUAU   very fine flour
ORGE   barley
SON   bran flour

Meats

ABATS   organ meats
AFRICAINE   with eggplant, mushrooms, potatoes and
   tomatoes
AGNEAU   lamb
AGNEAU, BARON D'   saddle and hind legs of lamb
AGNEAU, CARRÉ D'   rack, rib chops or cutlets of lamb
AGNEAU, CÔTELETTE D'   cutlet or lamb chop
AGNEAU: PRÉ-SALÉ   salt-marsh lamb
AGNEAU, ÉPAULE D'   shoulder of lamb
AGNEAU, FILET MIGNON   small, boned cutlet of lamb
AGNEAU, GIGOT D'   leg of lamb
AGNEAU DE LAIT   milk-fed lamb
AGNEAU, MÉDAILLON D'   small, boned cutlet of lamb
AGNEAU, NOISETTE D'   small, boned, finest cut cutlet of
   lamb
AGNEAU PERSILLÉ   baked leg of lamb larded with pork
   fat, garlic, wine, parsley
AGNEAU, POITRINE D'   breast of lamb
AGNEAU, SELLE D'   saddle of lamb
ALLEMANDE   with noodles and mashed potatoes
ALOSE ADOUR   herring stuffed and baked with ham
ALOUETTE SANS TÊTE   sliced veal rolled and stuffed
   with meat
ALOYAU   sirloin of beef

ALSACIENNE   with sauerkraut, ham and sausages

AMOURETTES   bone marrow of calf or ox

ANDALOUSE   with green peppers, eggplant and tomatoes

ANTIBOISE, À L'   with cheese, garlic, tomatoes and sardines or anchovy or tuna

ARCHIDUC   with cream and paprika

ARIÉGEOISE   with cabbage, pork, potatoes, beans

ARLÉSIENNE   with eggplant, olives, onions, potatoes, rice and tomatoes

ARTICHAUT À LA BARIGOULE   artichoke stuffed with meat or mushroom and salted pork

ASPIC DE VEAU   veal in aspic

ASSIETTE ANGLAISE   platter of assorted cold cuts or cold meats

ASSIETTE CHARCUTERIE   plate of dried sausage and pâté

ASSIETTE DE VIANDES FROIDES   cold cuts of meat

ATTEREAUX   deep fried vegetables or meat with sauce

AUBERGINE FARCIE ARMÉNIENNE   baked eggplant stuffed with lamb

BAECKENOFE   beef, mutton, pork stewed in wine and potatoes

BARON   hindquarters and legs of lamb

BASQUAISE   with ham and tomatoes or red peppers

BAVETTE   skirt steak

BEAUHARNAIS   tournedos in bearnaise sauce with artichoke hearts, potato balls and mushrooms

BEIGNET SOUFFLÉ   fritter with fish or meat filling

BELLE COMTOISE   veal with crumbs, baked with cheese and ham

BESI   beef jerky

BIFTECK   beefsteak

BIFTECK À L'ALLEMANDE   hamburger

BIFTECK À L'HAMBOURGEOISE   hamburger

BIFTECK AU POIVRE   pepper steak

BIFTECK MARCHAND DE VIN   steak sautéed with red wine

BITOK   ground beef and onions in croquette shape

BITOKE   French hamburger

BLANQUETTE   veal, lamb, chicken, seafood in white sauce

BLANQUETTE D'AGNEAU   lamb stew with mushrooms and onions

BLANQUETTE DE VEAU   veal stew with onions and mushrooms

BLANQUETTE DE VEAU À L'ANCIENNE   veal cutlets sautéed with onions, carrots, mushrooms, heavy cream

BLEU, AU   blood rare, usually for steak

BOEUF   beef

BOEUF À L'ARLÉSIENNE   beef stewed with tomatoes, eggplant, onions and olive oil

BOEUF BOUILLI   boiled beef

BOEUF BOURGUIGNON   beef stewed with red wine, onions and mushrooms

BOEUF BRAISÉ   braised beef

BOEUF EN DAUBE   marinated beef stewed in wine and vegetables

BOEUF GROS SEL   boiled beef with vegetables and coarse salt

BOEUF MIROTON   sautéed and baked beef with tomato sauce and sour pickles

BOEUF MODE EN GELÉE   jellied braised beef

BOEUF SALÉ   corned beef or salt beef

BOEUF, BAVETTE DE   skirt or flank steak

BOHÉMIENNE   with fried potatoes, olives, mushrooms

BOITELLE   cooked with mushrooms

BONNE FEMME   garnish of bacon, potatoes, mushrooms and onions

BOUC   male goat

BOUCHÉE À LA FINANCIÈRE   chicken and lambs' brains in creamy, sherry sauce

BOUDIN BLANC QUERCYNOIS   white pudding made with chicken and veal

BOUILLI   boiled

BOULETTE   meatball or fishball

BOURGEOISE, À LA   braised meat, family style

BOURGUIGNONNE, À LA   with red wine, onions, mushrooms and bacon

BREBIS   sheep

BRESI   dried, smoked beef in thin slices

BROCHETTE   meat or fish and vegetables on a skewer

BROCHETTE JURASSIENNE   pieces of cheese wrapped in ham and fried

BROUFADE   beef and onion stew with anchovies and capers

CABRI   kid goat

CACHUSE   braised pork

CAILLETTE   pork liver and bacon croquette

CAION   pork

CANNELON   puff-pastry with meat or fish filling

CAPILOTADE   meat hash

CARBONADE   braised beef stew with beer and onions

CARBONADE DE BOEUF PROVENÇALE   casserole of beef, onions and potatoes

CARBONADE FLAMANDE   browned slices of beef cooked in beer

CARRÉ   rack

CARRÉ D'AGNEAU   rack of lamb

CARRÉ D'AGNEAU PERSILLÉ   roast lamb with parsley

CARRÉ DE PORC   rack of pork

CARRÉ DE PORC RÔTI   roast loin of pork

CARRÉ DE VEAU   rack of veal

CASSOULET   casserole of beans, sausages, duck, pork, lamb

CASSOULET DE CASTELNAUDARY   white bean stew with goosefat, lamb, pork

CASSOULET PÉRIGOURDIN   stew of beans, mutton and sausage

CASSOULET TOULOUSAIN   stew of beans, onion, pork, lamb, sausage, duck or goose

CATALANE   eggplant, tomatoes, onions, peppers and rice

CATALANE, MOUTON À LA   mutton braised in wine with ham, vegetables and garlic

CAUCHOISE   white meat in cream with Calvados sauce and apples

CERVELLES   brains of calf or lamb

CERVELLES AU BEURRE NOIR   sautéed brains in brown butter sauce

CÉVÉNOLE   with chestnuts and mushrooms

CHABLISIENNE   cooked and served in white wine

CHACHLIK   lamb or beef roasted on a skewer with onions and peppers

CHAIR   fleshy portion of either poultry or meat

CHAMPENOISE (POTÉE)   stew of ham, sausage and cabbage

CHARCUTERIE ASSORTIE   assorted pork products

CHÂTEAU ENTRECÔTE   thick sirloin steak

CHÂTEAUBRIAND   thick filet steak

CHEVREAU   young goat

CHILIENNE   with rice and sweet peppers

CHOU FARCI   stuffed cabbage

COCHON   pig

COCHON DE LAIT   suckling pig

COCHON DE LAIT EN GELÉE   suckling pig in aspic

COEUR   heart

COEUR FILET   choice cut of steak

COLLET   mutton neck or veal

CONFIT   duck, goose, or pork preserved in its own fat

CONTRE-FILET   slice of steak

CORDON BLEU, ESCALOPE   veal with ham and cheese

CORNET   slice of ham or tongue rolled and stuffed; also an ice cream cone

CÔTE   chop; rib

CÔTE D'AGNEAU   lamb chops

CÔTE DE BOEUF   rib steak

CÔTE DE PORC   pork chop

CÔTE DE VEAU   veal chop

CÔTE DE VEAU EN PAPILLOTE   veal chops baked in a parchment bag with mushrooms, onion, parsley and butter

CÔTELETTE   chop

CÔTELETTE D'AGNEAU   lamb cutlet

CÔTELETTE D'AGNEAU CHAMPVALLON lamb chops baked in onions and potatoes

CÔTELETTES DE PORC AUX PRUNEAUX pork cutlets with prunes

CÔTELETTES DE PORC HERBS pork chops with herbs

CÔTELETTES NIVERNAISE casserole of veal or pork chops baked with carrots, potatoes and artichoke hearts

CÔTES DE BOEUF RÔTI roast beef ribs

CÔTES DE PORC À L'AUVERGNATE baked pork chops with cabbage

CÔTES DE VEAU À L'ARDENNAISE braised veal chops and ham

CÔTES DE VEAU À LA BONNE FEMME veal chops sautéed with onions and butter

CÔTES DE VEAU AUX HERBES veal chops with herbs

COUSCOUS semolina or hard wheat flour, usually served with a spicy lamb or chicken stew

COUSINAT stew made of ham, artichokes, carrots and green beans

CRÉOLE with rice, sweet peppers and tomatoes

CRETONS fat crisps

CROQUE-MONSIEUR toasted or fried cheese and ham sandwich

CROQUETTE ground meat, fish, fowl or vegetables, coated in breadcrumbs and deep fried

CROÛTE in pastry

CUISSEAU leg of veal

CUISSOT DE PORC RÔTI roast leg of pork

CULOTTE beef rump

DAGH KEBAB veal, onions and tomatoes grilled on a skewer

DAUBE beef stew with red wine

DAUBE DE BOEUF PROVENÇALE casserole of beef with wine and vegetables

DAUBE MORETON mutton stew prepared with herbs and vegetables

DAUBE PROVENÇALE beef stew mushrooms and onions in red wine

DEFARDE   stew of tripe and lambs' feet

DIABLE   very spicy, peppery sauce

ÉCHINE   spare ribs

ÉMINCÉ   very thin slice of meat

ENDIVE BRUXELLOISE   steamed endive rolled in ham

ENTRECÔTE   beef rib steak

ENTRECÔTE CHASSEUR   steak with tomato sauce, shallots and wine

ENTRECÔTE CHÂTEAU   large thick steak

ENTRECÔTE MAÎTRE D'HÔTEL   beef rib steak with herb butter

ENTRECÔTE MARCHAND DE VIN   beef steak with wine sauce

ENTRECÔTE MINUTE   thin steak

ÉPAULE   shoulder

ÉPAULE D'AGNEAU FARCIE   stuffed shoulder of lamb

ÉPAULE DE VEAU   shoulder of veal

ÉPIGRAMMES D'AGNEAU ST. GERMAIN   breast of lamb with peas

ESCALOPES   thin slices of meat

ESCALOPES À LA VIENNOISE   breaded veal cutlet

ESCALOPES DE VEAU   slices of veal

ESCALOPES DE VEAU À LA CRÈME   sliced veal with cream sauce

ESCALOPES DE VEAU BELLE COMTOISE   baked veal with cheese and ham

ESCALOPES DE VEAU GRATINÉES   casserole of veal with ham and cheese

ESCALOPES DE VEAU HOLSTEIN   veal cutlet topped with fried egg

ESCALOPES DE VEAU SAUTÉES À L'ESTRAGON   sautéed veal with tarragon

ESTOMAC   sheep stomach

ESTOUFFADE   stew of beef, pork, onions, mushrooms and wine

ESTOUFFADE DE BOEUF   beef with onions, wine, bacon

ESTOUFFAT   meat stewed with wine, vegetables and pork

ESTOUFFAT DE HARICOTS   stew of sausages or ham, white beans and pork

FAGOT   meatball

FAGOUE   sweetbreads

FAUX-FILET   sirloin steak

FECHUN   stuffed cabbage

FERMIÈRE, À LA   braised meat with vegetables

FILET   boneless cut of meat

FILET DE BOEUF   fillet of beef

FILET DE BOEUF CROÛTÉ   fillet of beef in pastry

FILET DE BOEUF RÔTI   roast fillet of beef

FILET DE PORC   pork fillet

FILET DE VEAU   veal fillet

FILET GRILLÉ   fillet steak

FILET MIGNON DE PORC NORMANDE   pork with apples in cider

FILETS MIGNONS DE BOEUF   small cuts of beef

FLAMMEKUECHE   tart with bacon, onions, cream cheese

FLANCHET DE BOEUF   flank steak

FOIE   liver

FOIE DE VEAU   calf's liver

FOIE DE VEAU À LA MOUTARDE   calf's liver with mustard and herbs

FOIE DE VEAU SAUTÉ   sautéed calf's liver

FOIE GRAS   goose liver

FORESTIÈRE   garnish of wild mushrooms, bacon and potatoes

FRESSURE   stew of pig's lung

FRIAND   meat patty

FRICADELLES   chopped meat patties, may have onion and potato, added to soups

FRICANDEAU   sliced veal braised with vegetables and wine

FRICASSÉE   meat, poultry or fish braised in wine or butter with cream

FRICASSÉE DE VEAU   veal stew

FRITONS   residue obtained by frying pork fat

FRITOT   small, deep fried pieces of beef, lamb, chicken or veal

FROMAGE DE PORC   jellied pork loaf
GALANTINE   boneless meat or poultry stuffed, cooked, sliced and served cold
GASCONNADE   roasted leg of mutton
GELÉE DE VIANDE   wine flavored meat jelly
GIBELOTTE   fricassee of rabbit in wine
GIBELOTTE DE LAPIN   rabbit stew with wine sauce
GIGORIT   pig's head in red wine
GIGOT   leg or haunch
GIGOT D'AGNEAU   roast leg of lamb
GIGOT D'AGNEAU À LA BOULANGÈRE   leg of lamb roasted with fried onions and potatoes
GIGOT D'AGNEAU RÔTI   roast leg of lamb on a spit
GIGOT DE MOUTON   leg of mutton
GIGOT FARCI, RÔTI À LA MOUTARDE   stuffed leg of lamb roasted in mustard glaze
GÎTE   shin of beef
GLACE DE VIANDE   meat glaze from stock
GORENFLOT   garnish of sausage, potatoes and cabbage
GOULASCH   beef stew with onions and paprika
GOULASCH VEAU   veal goulash
GOURMANDISES   sweet meats
GRAISSE NORMANDE   pork and beef fat used for cooking
GRAS-DOUBLE   baked tripe with onions and wine
GRASSET   cut of beef
GRATIN (AU)   dish with a browned cheese and crusty breadcrumb topping over cream sauce
GRATIN LANDAIS   potato, ham and cheese dish
GRATTONS   crisp fried pork, goose, or duck skin
GRENADIN   small veal scallop
GRENADINS DE BOEUF   beef cooked with vegetables, wine, onions and mushrooms
GRIGNAUDES   fried pieces of pork
GRILLADE   grilled meat
GRILLETTES   bits of fat grilled till crispy
HACHIS   minced or chopped meat or fish, like hash
HACHIS DE BOEUF   minced beef

HACHIS PARMENTIER   shepherd's pie of minced meat in sauce

HACHUA   ham stewed with peppers and onions

HARICOT DE MOUTON   stew, with mutton and white beans

HOCHEPOT   thick stew, usually oxtail

HONGROISE, À L'   with paprika and cream

HURE DE PORC   pig's head in jelly

JAMBON   ham

JAMBON À LA BAYONNAISE   ham with sausage, mushrooms, tomatoes and rice

JAMBON À LA CRÈME   ham in cream sauce

JAMBON AU CIDRE   ham cooked in cider

JAMBON AURORE   cooked ham in a butter, cream, tomato sauce

JAMBON BLANC   boiled ham

JAMBON BRAISÉ   braised ham in sherry wine

JAMBON CRU   raw cured ham

JAMBON CUIT   cooked ham

JAMBON D'AUVERGNE   raw, dried, salt cured smoked ham

JAMBON D'YORK   smoked English ham, often poached

JAMBON DE BAYONNE   cured ham in thin slices

JAMBON DE BOURGOGNE   cold cooked ham in gelatin

JAMBON DE CAMPAGNE   country smoked ham

JAMBON DE MONTAGNE   country smoked ham mountain style

JAMBON DE PARIS   cooked ham

JAMBON DE PARME   smoked ham eaten raw in paper-thin slices, prosciutto ham

JAMBON DE WESTPHALIE   German Westphalian ham, raw-cured and smoked

JAMBON DU PAYS   country ham, usually salt cured

JAMBON EN CROÛTE   ham in pastry

JAMBON FOIN   ham simmered in water with herbs

JAMBON FROID   cold ham

JAMBON FUMÉ   smoked ham

JAMBON, L'OS DE   ham bone in
JAMBON MADÈRE   ham prepared with a Madeira wine
JAMBON PERSILLÉ   cold preserved ham in gelatin
JAMBON POCHÉ   ham poached in stock
JAMBON SALÉ   salt cured ham
JAMBON SAUPIQUET   ham in wine and cream sauce
JAMBON SEC   dried ham
JAMBONNEAU   cured ham shank
JAMBONNETTE   boned and stuffed knuckle of ham
JARRET   knuckle
JARRET DE BOEUF EN DAUBE   shin of beef stewed with
   wine in a casserole
JARRET DE PORC SALÉ   salted shin of pork
JARRET DE VEAU   veal shin
JARRET DE VEAU AU CITRON   stewed knuckle of veal
   with lemon
JULIENNE   slivered vegetables or meat
KASSLER   rolled pork fillet
KEBAB   meat cooked on a skewer
KIG HA FARS   slow cooked meat and vegetable casserole
LAME   very thin slice
LANDAISE   cooked in garlic and onions with goose fat
LANGUE   tongue
LANGUE À L'ÉCARLATE   salted tongue
LANGUE D'AGNEAU BRAISÉE AUX PETITS, POIS
   braised lamb tongue
LANGUE DE BOEUF   ox tongue
LANGUE DE BOEUF BRAISÉE AU MADÈRE   beef
   tongue braised in Madeira sauce
LANGUE DE VEAU   calf's tongue
LANGUE FOURRÉE   stuffed tongue
LANGUIER   smoked pork tongue
LAPEREAU   young rabbit
LAPIN   rabbit
LAPIN À LA HAVRAISE   roast rabbit with bacon in
   cream sauce
LARD   bacon

LARD DE POITRINE FUMÉ   smoked bacon slab
LARDONS   cubes of fried bacon
LEBERKNEPFEN   calf's liver dumplings
LÈCHE   thin slice of bread or meat
LEWERKNOPFLES   liver dumplings
LIÉGEOISE   made with juniper berries and gin
LONGE   loin
LONGE DE VEAU   loin of veal
LORRAINE, À LA   braised in wine
LYONNAISE, À LA   garnished with onions; in the style of
   Lyons
MARINÉ   marinated
MÉDAILLON   a small, circular cut of meat or poultry
MÉDAILLON DE VEAU   miniature veal steak
MENON   roast goat
MERGUEZ   small spicy sausage
MIROTON   stew of meats flavored with onions
MIROTON, BOEUF   sliced boiled beef in onion and sour
   pickle sauce sprinkled with cheese
MOELLE   beef bone marrow
MOUSSAKA   a Greek lamb and eggplant dish
MOUSSE   beaten egg whites or whipped cream; meat,
   poultry or fish finely ground and served in a mold
MOUTON   mutton
MOUTON AUX PISTACHES   mutton braised in wine
   with garlic, vegetables and pistachio nuts
MUSEAU DE PORC   vinegared pork muzzle or snout
NAGE, À LA   cooked and served in bouillon poaching
   liquid
NAVARIN   lamb or mutton stew with potatoes and onions
NAVARIN AUX POMMES   mutton stew with potatoes
   and tomatoes
NAVARIN D'AGNEAU   brown lamb stew
NAVARIN DE MOUTON   roasted mutton stew with
   consommé, onions, cloves, potatoes
NAVARIN PRINTANIER   lamb stew with carrots, onions,
   potatoes, turnips, green peas and beans

NIÇOISE, À LA   refers to dishes with onions, garlic, olive oil, tomatoes, anchovies

NOISETTE D'AGNEAU   lamb cutlet from the fillet

NOISETTE D'AGNEAU CLAMART   lamb, artichoke hearts and peas

NOIX DE VEAU   center cut of veal

NORMANDE, À LA   fish or meat cooked with apple cider; apple dessert with cream

OISEAUX SANS TÊTES   pieces of meat rolled up and stuffed with varying ingredients

OREILLES DE PORC   cooked pig's ears, served grilled with a coating of egg and bread crumbs

OS À LA MOELLE   marrow bone

PACARET   made with sherry

PAILLARDE, VEAU   grilled boneless veal steak or cutlet

PALERON   shoulder of beef

PALERON DE BOEUF   chuck or pot roast

PANÉ   prepared with breadcrumbs

PANTIN   pastry filled with ground pork

PAPILLOTE, EN   cooked in parchment paper or foil envelope

PARMESANÉ   prepared with parmesan cheese

PÂTÉ   minced meat molded, spiced, baked in pastry, served in slices hot or cold

PÂTÉ DE BIFTECK   beefsteak pie

PÂTÉ DE FOIE GRAS   goose liver

PÂTÉ EN CROÛTE AUX ÉPINARDS   veal, ham and pork pie with spinach

PAUPIETTE   slice of chicken, fish or meat filled with another mixture, rolled up and sautéed

PAUPIETTE DE VEAU   slice of veal, usually filled with a mixture and rolled

PETIT SALÉ   salt pork

PETIT SALÉ AUX LENTILLES   boiled bacon with lentils in a casserole

PIED   foot

PIED DE COCHON   pig's foot

PIED DE MOUTON   stuffed sheep's foot

PIED DE PORC   pig's foot
PIED DE PORC SAINTE-MENEHOULD   grilled pig feet
PIED DE VEAU   calves' feet
PLAT DE CÔTES   boiled beef short ribs and vegetables
PLAT DE CÔTES DE PORC RÔTIES   roast spare ribs
POINT, À   medium rare steak or ripe
POITRINE   breast of meat or poultry
POITRINE DE MOUTON   breast of mutton
POITRINE DE MOUTON FARCIE   mutton breast stuffed
   with ham
POITRINE DE VEAU   breast of veal
POITRINE FUMÉE   smoked bacon
POMPONNETTE   ground meat or poultry in a pastry case
PORC   pork
PORC, CARRÉ DE   rib roast of pork
PORC, CÔTE DE   loin chop of pork
PORC, ÉCHINE DE   pork spare rib
PORC MARENGO   pork stewed with wine and tomatoes
PORC, PLAT DE CÔTE DE   spare ribs
PORCELET   young suckling pig
POT-AU-FEU À LA NORMANDE   boiled dinner of beef,
   pork, veal or chicken, with vegetables
POTÉE BOURGUIGNONNE   thick stew of vegetables,
   pork and sausage
POTÉE CHAMPENOISE   stew of ham, bacon, sausage
   and cabbage
POTÉE LIMOUSINE   stew made of pork, chestnuts and
   red cabbage
POTÉE LORRAINE   stew of pork, sausage, cabbage
POULET RÔTI   roast chicken
PRÉ-SALÉ   distinctive tasting salt marsh lamb
QUENELLE   dumpling, usually of veal, fish or poultry
QUEUE DE BOEUF   oxtail
QUEUE DE BOEUF FARCIE   stuffed oxtail
QUICHE   tart with egg and cream, meat or vegetable filling
RAGOÛT   stew, usually of meat
REGUIGNEU   fried country ham

RILLETTE DE LAPIN   mince of pork and rabbit
RILLETTE DE TOURS   ground up pork meat, somewhat
   coarser than pâté
RILLETTES DE PORC   soft potted pork
RIS D'AGNEAU   lamb sweetbreads
RIS D'AGNEAU BRAISÉ   braised lamb sweetbreads
RIS DE VEAU   veal sweetbreads
RIS DE VEAU À LA CRÈME   braised sweetbreads in cream
RIS DE VEAU AU BEURRE NOIR   sweetbreads in brown
   butter sauce
RIS DE VEAU GUIZOT   braised sweetbreads
RISSOLE   ground mixture covered with pastry and deep fried
ROGNON   kidney
ROGNON BLANC   testicle
ROGNON DE MOUTON   sheep kidney
ROGNON DE VEAU   veal kidney
ROGNON DE VEAU À LA LIÉGOISE   calf's kidneys,
   juniper berries and gin
ROGNON DE VEAU EN CASSEROLE   kidney in butter
   and mustard sauce
ROGNON DE VEAU FLAMBÉ   sautéed kidney flambéed
   with mushroom sauce
ROGNON EN BROCHETTE   lambs kidneys on a skewer
ROGNON EN CASSEROLE   sautéed kidneys with mus-
   tard sauce
ROGNON SAUTÉ FLAMBÉ   veal and lamb kidney,
   sautéed and flambéed
ROGNON SAUTÉ MADÈRE   sautéed kidney with wine
ROGNONNADE   veal loin with kidneys attached
ROMSTECK   rump steak
ROSBIF   roast beef
RÔTI   roast
RÔTI DE BOEUF JARDINIÈRE   roast beef with vegetables
RÔTI DE BOEUF POÊLÉ MATIGNON   roast beef with
   vegetables and potatoes
RÔTI, FILET   roasted fillet
RÔTI, FOIE   roasted liver

RÔTI, JARRET   roasted knuckle
RÔTI, ROGNON   roasted kidneys
ROUELLE DE VEAU   veal shank
RUMSTECK   rumpsteck
SAIGNANT   rare steak
SALPICON   diced vegetables, meat and/or fish in a sauce
SAUTÉ, BOEUF   beef cooked in red wine and tomatoes
SAUTÉ DE PORC AUX CHAMPIGNONS   pork sautéed
   with mushrooms
SAUTÉ DE VEAU   veal browned lightly in fat
SAUTÉ DE VEAU AUX CHAMPIGNONS   veal sautéed
   with mushrooms
SCHIFELA   pork with pickled turnips
SELLE D'AGNEAU RÔTIE À LA PERSILLADE   roast
   saddle of lamb with parsley
SOUFFLÉ REINE   soufflé of poultry or meat
STEAK   steak
STEAK À POINT   cooked medium steak
STEAK AU FOUR   steak baked with herbs
STEAK BIEN CUIT   well-done steak
STEAK DIANE   steak sautéed with wine and peppercorns
STEAK HACHÉ   hamburger steak
STEAK MAÎTRE D'HÔTEL   grilled or pan-fried steak
STEAK POIVRÉ   steak with crushed peppercorns
STEAK SAIGNANT   very rare steak
STEAK SAUTÉ HENRI IV   filet steaks with artichokes or
   mushrooms, Bearnaise sauce
STEAK TARTARE   raw steak, chopped onions, capers,
   worcestire sauce and raw egg served on top
SURLONGE   sirloin
TAGINE   spicy stew of veal, lamb, chicken and vegetables
TENDRONS DE VEAU   braised veal
TERRINE   earthenware container for baking meat, game,
   fish or vegetable mixture
TERRINE DE BOEUF   beef stew with vegetables and wine
TERRINE DE FOIE   liver cooked in an earthenware
   container

TERRINE DE JAMBON   finely ground ham, combined with cream and sherry

TERRINE DE MOUTON   finely ground mutton combined with spices and cream

TERRINE DE PORC   pork pâté with ham

TERRINE DE VEAU   veal pâté with ham

TÊTE DE VEAU   calf's head

TÊTE DE VEAU À LA VINAIGRETTE   calf's head served in oil and vinegar

TIMBALE DE JAMBON   molded ham custard

TORTUE   turtle, tortoise

TOURNEDOS   center of beef fillet, grilled or sautéed

TOURNEDOS À LA BÉARNAISE   grilled steak served on toast with bearnaise sauce

TOURNEDOS À LA PÉRIGOURDINE   cuts of steak with truffles

TOURNEDOS ALEXANDRA   steak sautéed with artichoke hearts

TOURNEDOS ARLÉSIEN   steak sautéed, served with fried eggplant and tomatoes

TOURNEDOS AUX CHAMPIGNONS   beef fillets with mushrooms

TOURNEDOS CHASSEUR   pan-fried steak in wine, mushrooms and tomato paste

TOURNEDOS CLAMART   pan-fried steak with fresh peas

TOURNEDOS DES GOURMETS   steak fried in sherry, served with goose liver

TOURNEDOS GRILLÉ   grilled steak

TOURNEDOS MAÎTRE D'HÔTEL   grilled or pan-fried steak

TOURNEDOS ROSSINI   sautéed tournedos garnished with liver and truffles

TOURTE DE MOUTON   mutton pie

TOURTE LORRAINE   tart with pork and veal in cream

TRANCHE DE JAMBON ROSE-MARIE   ham slices in cream sauce

TRIPE   stomach lining of a cow

TRIPE À LA MODE DE CAEN   beef tripe, onions, leeks, cooked in cider and Calvados brandy
TRIPE FERTÉ-MACÉ   tripe cooked on skewers
TRIPOUX   mutton tripe
VEAU   veal
VEAU À LA FLAMANDE   veal braised with fruits
VEAU BLANQUETTE DE   veal stew
VEAU CUSTINE   fried veal chops with tomato sauce
VEAU, FRICADELLES DE   ground veal patties
VEAU HOLSTEIN   sautéed veal with fried eggs and anchovies
VEAU, JARRET DE   veal shank
VEAU, POITRINE DE   stuffed breast of veal
VEAU, RIS DE   veal sweetbreads
VEAU RÔTI   roast veal
VEAU, SAUTÉ DE   veal stew
VEAU SYLVIE   veal roasted with ham and cheese
VEAU, TENDRON DE   breast of veal stewed with vegetables
VIANDE   meat
VIANDE CHAUDE   hot meat
VIANDE FROIDE   cold meat
VIANDE SÉCHÉE   cured dried beef
ZINGARA   with tomato, ham and mushrooms

Pasta

BAGRATION   macaroni and artichoke hearts, with tomato, mayonnaise and eggs
CHEVEUX D'ANGE   very fine pasta, like angelhair
LASAGNE   baked pasta and cheese with meat sauce
NOUILLES   noodles
NOUILLES AU FROMAGE   noodles with cheese
PARMESANÉ   prepared with parmesan cheese
PÂTES ALIMENTAIRES   spaghetti, macaroni
SPAETZLE   small noodle dumplings
TOTELOTS   hot noodle salad
VERMICELLE   very thin spaghetti

Pâté

BROCCANA   sausage-meat and veal pâté
HURE DE SAUMON   pâté prepared with salmon
MERLE   blackbird pâté
PÂTÉ ARDENNAIS   pork and seasonings in pastry
PÂTÉ D'AMANDES   almond paste
PÂTÉ D'ANGUILLE   eel pâté
PÂTÉ DE BÉCASSE   woodcock pâté
PÂTÉ D'OIE   goose pâté
PÂTÉ DE CAMPAGNE   pork pâté
PÂTÉ DE CANARD   duck pâté
PÂTÉ DE CHEVREUIL   venison pâté
PÂTÉ DE FOIE   liver pâté
PÂTÉ DE FOIE DE PORC   finely ground pork livers
PÂTÉ DE FOIE DE VOLAILLE   chicken liver pâté
PÂTÉ DE GIBIER   pâté made with game
PÂTÉ DE GRIVE   pâté made with thrush or songbird
PÂTÉ DE LAPIN   rabbit pâté
PÂTÉ DE LIÈVRE   pâté of wild hare
PÂTÉ DE POISSON   fish pâté
PÂTÉ DE TÊTE   pâté made from calf's head
PÂTÉ EN CROÛTE   mixture covered with pastry
PÂTÉ EN CROÛTE AUX ÉPINARDS   veal, ham and pork
   pie with spinach
PÂTÉ MAISON   house specialty
PETIT PÂTÉ   small pastry filled with ground meat
RILLETTE   soft, spreadable pork or goose paste
SAUCISSE, TIMBALE DE   sausage pâté in crust
TERRINE AUX AROMATES   herb pâté
TERRINE DE GIBIER   wild game pâté
TERRINE DE LAPIN   rabbit pâté
TERRINE DE PORC   pork pâté with ham
TERRINE DE VEAU   veal pâté with ham

Potatoes

ALIGOT   mashed potatoes with fresh Cantal cheese and garlic

ALLUMETTES fried shoestring potatoes or pastry strips

BOUCHÉE DUCHESSE mashed potatoes with mushrooms and creamed chicken, baked

CHÂTEAU POMMES potatoes cooked in butter

CRÊPES DE POMMES DE TERRE grated potato pancakes

DAUPHINOIS, GRATIN potatoes cooked with milk and cheese

DUCHESSE, POMMES DE TERRE dish containing creamed or mashed potatoes

FLOUTES potato balls

GALETTE DE POMMES DE TERRE potato pancake

GALETTE LYONNAISE mashed potatoes and onions

GNOCCHI potato and flour dumpling

GRATIN DAUPHINOIS scalloped potatoes

GRATIN DE POMMES DE TERRE SAUCISSON sausage and potato casserole

GRATIN LANDAIS potato, ham and cheese dish

GRATIN SAVOYARD casserole of potatoes, bouillon, cheese and butter

IRLANDAISE, À L' served with potatoes

LAITANCE SABOT baked potatoes stuffed with herring roe

MATAFAN thick potato pancake

OULADE stew made from potatoes, cabbage, sausage and pork

PARMENTIER dish with potatoes

PATATE sweet potato

POMMES DE TERRE potatoes

POMMES DE TERRE À L'AIL potatoes puréed with garlic

POMMES DE TERRE À L'AIL PURÉE DE garlic mashed potatoes

POMMES DE TERRE À L'ANGLAISE boiled potatoes

POMMES DE TERRE À L'HUILE French potato salad, with vinegar, olive oil, herbs

POMMES DE TERRE À LA BOULANGÈRE potatoes cooked with meat

POMMES DE TERRE À LA LYONNAISE sautéed potatoes with onions

POMMES DE TERRE À LA SARLADAISE   casserole of potatoes cooked in goose fat

POMMES DE TERRE ALLUMETTES   shoestring potatoes

POMMES DE TERRE ANNA   sliced potatoes baked in butter

POMMES DE TERRE AU GRATIN DAUPHINOIS   baked scalloped potatoes

POMMES DE TERRE BASQUAISE   baked potatoes, stuffed with ham, tomatoes and garlic

POMMES DE TERRE BIGOUDENN   baked slices of unpeeled potato

POMMES DE TERRE BOUILLIES   boiled potatoes

POMMES DE TERRE BRETONNE   potatoes with cream, celery and onions

POMMES DE TERRE BYRON   baked potato pancake

POMMES DE TERRE CHATOUILLARD   deep-fried ribbon potatoes

POMMES DE TERRE: CHIPS   potato chips

POMMES DE TERRE, COLLERETTES DE   thin slices of potato, fried

POMMES DE TERRE CROQUETTES DE   mashed, deep-fried in breadcrumbs

POMMES DE TERRE DAUPHINE   fried balls of mashed potatoes mixed with pastry

POMMES DE TERRE DAUPHINOISE   baked sliced potatoes, milk, garlic and cheese

POMMES DE TERRE DUCHESSE   mashed potatoes with butter, egg yolks and nutmeg

POMMES DE TERRE EN PAILLE   fried julienned potatoes

POMMES DE TERRE EN ROBE DES CHAMPS   potatoes cooked with skins on

POMMES DE TERRE FRITES   french fried potatoes

POMMES DE TERRE GRATINÉES   potatoes browned with cheese

POMMES DE TERRE LORETTE   fried potato croquettes

POMMES DE TERRE MACAIRE   baked mashed potatoes fried in flat cakes

POMMES DE TERRE MAÎTRE D'HÔTEL boiled potatoes, sautéed with hot milk

POMMES DE TERRE MONT-DORÉ mashed potatoes and cheese baked in the oven

POMMES DE TERRE, MOUSSELINE DE puréed with butter, egg yolks and cream

POMMES DE TERRE NATURE plain boiled potatoes

POMMES DE TERRE PARISIENNE fried potato balls

POMMES DE TERRE PARMENTIER large cubes of potatoes sautéed in butter

POMMES DE TERRE PONT-NEUF classic fries

POMMES DE TERRE PURÉE DE mashed potatoes

POMMES DE TERRE RISSOLÉES sautéed potatoes

POMMES DE TERRE SAVOYARDE AU GRATIN sliced potatoes baked with cheese

POMMES DE TERRE SOUFFLÉES slices of potato fried twice to fluff up

POMMES DE TERRE ST. FLOUR sliced potatoes with bacon baked on cabbage leaves

POMMES DE TERRE VAPEUR steamed or boiled potatoes

POMMES DE TERRE VOISIN potato cake of sliced potato and cheese

POMMES DE TERRE YVETTE baked potato strips

RÂPÉE À LA MORVANDELLE grated potato baked with eggs and cheese

TARTOUFFE potato

TROUFFE slang for potato

TRUFFADE fried potato mashed with cheese, tomatoes, bacon and garlic

TRUFFIAT potato cake

Poultry

ABATTIS giblets of fowl

AFRICAINE with eggplant, mushrooms, potatoes and tomatoes

AIGUILLETTE DE CANETON   breast of duckling strips
AILE   wing of poultry or game bird
AILERON   wing tip
ALICOT   fowl wings and giblets stewed with chestnuts (Périgord)
ALLEMANDE   with noodles and mashed potatoes
ANTIBOISE, À L'   with cheese, garlic, tomatoes and sardines or anchovy or tuna
ARCHIDUC   with cream and paprika
ARIÉGEOISE   with cabbage, pork, potatoes, beans
ARLÉSIENNE   with eggplant, olives, onions, potatoes, rice and tomatoes
BALLOTTINE   poultry, boned, stuffed and rolled
BARBOTÉ   duck
BLANC DE VOLAILLE   boned breast of fowl
BLANQUETTE   veal, lamb, chicken, seafood in white sauce
BOHÉMIENNE   with fried potatoes, olives, mushrooms
BOITELLE   cooked with mushrooms
BOUDIN BLANC QUERCYNOIS   white pudding made with chicken and veal
BOURIBOT   spicy duck stew with red wine
CANARD   duck
CANARD À L'ORANGE   roast duck braised with oranges and orange liqueur
CANARD AUX CERISES   duck with cherries
CANARD AUX OLIVES   duck cooked with olives
CANARD MONTMORENCY   duck in wine flavored jelly with cherries
CANARD NANTAIS   delicate flavored small duck
CANARD ROUEN   cross between domestic and wild duck
CANARD ROUENNAIS   duck with sauce from the blood
CANARD VERT POIS   steamed duckling with peas
CANETON   duckling
CANETON À L'ORANGE   duckling with orange
CANETON À LA BIGARADE   duckling with bitter oranges
CANETON AUX CERISES   duckling with cherries
CANETON AUX NAVETS   duck with turnips

CANETON AUX OLIVES   duck with olives

CANETON MONTMORENCY   roast duck with poached cherries in a port sauce

CASSOULET   casserole of beans, sausages, duck, pork, and lamb

CASSOULET DE CASTELNAUDARY   white bean stew with goosefat, lamb, pork

CATALANE   eggplant, tomatoes, onions, peppers and rice

CÉLESTINE, POULARDE   sautéed chicken and mushrooms in wine, cream sauce

CÉVÉNOLE   with chestnuts and mushrooms

CHABLISIENNE   cooked and served in white wine

CHAIR   fleshy portion of either poultry or meat

CHAIR BLANCHE   white meat

CHAPON   capon or castrated chicken

CHAPON GROS SEL   capon baked in rock salt

CHAUD-FROID   poultry dish served cold with a sauce

CHILIENNE   with rice and sweet peppers

CONFIT   duck, goose, or pork preserved in its own fat

CONFIT D'OIE   goose preserved in its own fat in earthen jars

CONFIT DE CANARD   pieces of duck cooked and preserved in earthen jars

COQ   chicken

COQ À LA BIÈRE   chicken cooked in beer

COQ AU RIESLING   chicken in white wine and cream sauce

COQ AU VIN   chicken stewed in wine sauce

COU D'OIE FARCI   stuffed goose neck

COUSCOUS   semolina or hard wheat flour, usually served with a spicy lamb or chicken stew

CRAPAUDINE   poultry split and grilled

CRÉOLE   with rice, sweet peppers and tomatoes

CRÊPE À LA VOLAILLE   chicken pancake

CRÊTE DE COQ   cock's comb

CROQUE-MADAME   toasted or fried cheese and chicken sandwich

CROQUETTE   ground meat, fish, fowl or vegetables, coated in breadcrumbs and deep fried

CROUSTADE DE VOLAILLE   pastry shells with a chicken mixture

CROÛTE   in pastry

CUISSE   leg and thigh of poultry

CUISSE DE POULET   chicken drumstick

DEMI-DEUIL POULARDE   poached chicken with truffles

DEMIDOFF   chicken with pureed vegetables

DIABLE   very spicy, peppery sauce

DINDE   turkey

DINDON AUX MARRONS   turkey stuffed with chestnuts, sausage meat, pork, brandy and baked

DINDON FARCI AUX MARRONS   turkey stuffed with chestnuts

DINDON RÔTI   roast turkey

DODINE   cold, boned stuffed duck

DODINE DE CANARD   duck stewed with onions

DODINE DE VOLAILLE   marinated chicken stuffed and braised

FAISAN NORMAND   casserole of pheasant with salt pork, butter, apples, sour cream, pepper, applejack

FARCE ÉVOCATION LABUFERA   rice, mushroom and chicken liver stuffing

FOIE AUX RAISINS   chicken liver cooked in wine with grapes

FOIE DE CANARD   preserved duck livers

FOIE DE POULET   chicken liver

FOIE DE VOLAILLE   chicken liver

FOIE DE VOLAILLE SAUTÉ MADÈRE   chicken liver sautéed in Madeira wine sauce

FOIE GRAS AUX RAISINS   goose liver with grapes

FRICASSÉE   meat, poultry or fish braised in wine or butter with cream

FRICASSÉE DE VOLAILLE ET D'ÉCREVISSES   chicken and crayfish stewed in cream and wine

FRITOT   small, deep fried pieces of beef, lamb, chicken or veal

GALANTINE   boneless meat or poultry stuffed, cooked, sliced and served cold

GELINOTTE   prairie chicken or grouse

GÉSIER   gizzard

GRAISSERONS   crisply fried pieces of duck or goose skin, may also refer to potted pork

GRATIN (AU)   dish with a browned cheese and crusty breadcrumb topping over cream sauce

GRATTONS   crisp fried pork, goose, or duck skin

GRILLETTES   bits of fat grilled till crispy

JAMBON D'OIE   breast of smoked goose like ham in taste

JAMBON DE CANARD   smoked breast of duck, like ham in taste

LANDAISE   cooked in garlic and onions with goose fat

LIÉGEOISE   made with juniper berries and gin

LORRAINE, À LA   braised in wine

LOU MAGRET   breast of fattened duck

MAGRET DE CANARD   breast of duck, grilled rare

MARINÉ   marinated

MÉDAILLON   a small, circular cut of meat or poultry

MEURETTE, VOLAILLE EN   chicken stew with red wine, onions, as coq au vin

MOUSSE   beaten egg whites or whipped cream; meat, poultry or fish finely ground and served in a mold

MOUSSE DE FOIE GRAS   ground goose livers with cream and whipped with truffles

MOUSSE DE VOLAILLE EN GELÉE   cold chicken, whipped, then served with aspic

NAGE, À LA   cooked and served in bouillon poaching liquid

NIÇOISE, À LA   refers to dishes with onions, garlic, olive oil, tomatoes, anchovies

OEUF MIRETTE   tart with a poached egg yolk and chicken in a cream sauce

OIE BRAISÉE AUX PRUNEAUX   braised goose with prune and liver stuffing

OIE EN DAUBE   goose, stewed with wine

OIE RÔTIE AUX PRUNEAUX   roast goose with prune stuffing

OISON   a young goose
OYONNADE   goose stewed in wine
PACARET   made with sherry
PANÉ   pepared with breadcrumbs
PARMESANÉ   prepared with parmesan cheese
PAUPIETTE   slice of chicken, fish or meat filled with
   another mixture, rolled up and sautéed
PERDRIX À LA CATALANE   partridge stew
PETIT POUSSIN   a very small chicken
POITRINE   breast of meat or poultry
POITRINE D'OIE FUMÉE   smoked goose breast
POMPONNETTE   ground meat or poultry in a pastry case
POULARDE   large roasting chicken
POULARDE À L'ÉCREVISSE   chicken with crayfish in
   wine and cream sauce
POULARDE AU RIESLING   coq au vin, made with white
   wine instead of red
POULARDE AU VINAIGRE   chicken, tomatoes, wine,
   vinegar and cream sauce
POULARDE BASQUAISE   chicken with peppers, mush-
   rooms, eggplant
POULARDE BAYONNAISE   roasting hen with onions
POULARDE CÉLESTINE   chicken with mushrooms in a
   wine and cream sauce
POULARDE CHEVALIÈRE   chicken in pastry with
   mushrooms
POULARDE DE BRESSE EN BRIOCHE   chicken baked in
   a yeast dough
POULARDE DEMI-DEUIL   chicken with truffles, sim-
   mered in broth with cream sauce
POULARDE DEMI-DÉSOSSÉE   half-boned chicken
POULARDE DERBY   chicken with rice, foie gras, truffles, wine
POULARDE EN CHEMISE   poached stuffed chicken
POULARDE LYONNAISE   stuffed chicken with truffles,
   vegetables
POULARDE MÈRE FILLIOUX   chicken with sausage and
   sweetbreads, cooked in a cream sauce

POULARDE PAYSANNE   chicken in sauce with vege–
tables, bacon and potatoes

POULARDE STRASBOURGEOISE   chicken breasts
stuffed with ground goose livers

POULE   hen, also see poulet and poularde

POULE AU POT   chicken in the pot, chicken soup

POULE AU POT HENRI IV   stuffed chicken cooked in wine

POULE IVOIRE   boiled fowl with cream sauce

POULET   chicken, also see poularde and poule

POULET À L'ARMAGNAC   chicken with white cream
sauce and Armagnac brandy

POULET À LA CASSEROLE   chicken sautéed in a skillet

POULET À LA CRÈME   chicken in cream sauce

POULET À LA NIÇOISE   chicken cooked with garlic,
saffron and tomatoes

POULET À LA PARISIENNE   sautéed chicken with
mashed potatoes in wine

POULET À LA ROUILLEUSE   chicken in wine and garlic
sauce

POULET ALEXANDRA   sautéed chicken with cream sauce

POULET AU VIN JAUNE   chicken in a cream sauce made
with wine

POULET BARBOUILLÉ   chicken in wine sauce

POULET BASQUAISE   chicken with tomatoes and sweet
peppers

POULET BEAULIEU   chicken in artichokes, potatoes and
wine sauce

POULET BOIVIN   sautéed chicken with artichokes

POULET BORDEAUX   chicken fried with tomatoes, wine
and mushrooms

POULET CHASSEUR   sautéed chicken with shallots and
tomato sauce

POULET COCOTTE   baked chicken with pork, onions,
potatoes, artichoke hearts, chicken broth

POULET COCOTTE BONNE FEMME   baked chicken
with potatoes and bacon

POULET COMPOTE   chicken stew

POULET DIJON   chicken sautéed with wine, Dijon style mustard, sour cream

POULET DUC   chicken sautéed with brandy in heavy cream and wine

POULET EN GELÉE   jellied tarragon chicken

POULET FARCI   chicken stuffed with ham, liver and cooked in soup

POULET FORESTIÈRE   chicken sautéed with mushrooms, potatoes and Madeira

POULET FRIT   fried chicken

POULET GRILLÉ À LA DIABLE   chicken broiled with mustard, herb and breadcrumbs

POULET GRILLE NATUREL   plain broiled chicken

POULET KATOFF   grilled chicken served on mashed potatoes

POULET KIEV   deep fried breast of chicken stuffed with seasoned butter

POULET MARENGO   chicken sautéed in olive oil, with mushrooms, tomatoes

POULET MATELOTE   chicken in red wine

POULET NEVA   chicken stuffed with ground chicken liver in aspic

POULET POCHÉ AU RIZ   boiled chicken with rice

POULET POCHÉ AUX AROMATES   chicken simmered in white wine and vegetables

POULET RÔTI À L'ESTRAGON   chicken with tarragon cream sauce

POULET RÔTI AU BEURRE   chicken roasted in butter

POULET SAUTÉ À LA BORDELAISE   sautéed chicken with artichoke hearts

POULET SAUTÉ ARLÉSIEN   fried chicken with eggplant in white wine

POULET SAUTÉ AU VIN BLANC   chicken in cream and white wine

POULET SAUTÉ PARMENTIER   chicken sautéed with potatoes in wine

POULET VALLÉE D'AUGE   chicken with apples

POUSSIN   baby chicken, also see poule, poulet, poularde
QUENELLE   dumpling, usually of veal, fish or poultry
REINE, À LA   with mince meat or fowl
RISSOLE   ground mixture covered with pastry and deep fried
SALMIS   stewlike preparation of game birds or poultry in wine
SALPICON DE VOLAILLE   diced turkey or chicken in white wine sauce
SARCELLE   teal, small duck
SAUCE SUPRÊME   thick chicken stock base
SOUFFLÉ REINE   souffle of poultry or meat
SUPRÊME   boneless breast of poultry or a fillet of fish
SUPRÊME DE VOLAILLE   chicken breasts poached in butter, wine and cream sauce
SUPRÉME DE VOLAILLE ÉCOSSAISE   chicken breasts with vegetables
TAGINE   spicy stew of veal, lamb, chicken and vegetables
TERRINE DE CANARD   duck cooked in an earthenware container
TERRINE DE FOIES DE VOLAILLE   chicken liver in an earthenware container
TERRINE DE VOLAILLE   chicken cooked in an earthenware container
TERRINE MAISON   mixture of chicken, goose livers or pork
TIMBALE DE FOIES DE VOLAILLE   chicken liver mold
TOURTE DE CANETON   duck baked in a pie
TOURTIÈRE   chicken pie
VOLAILLE   poultry, also see poulet
VOLAILLE FROIDE   cold poultry
WATERZOOI   chicken or fish stew in creamy sauce
ZINGARA   with tomato, ham and mushrooms

Quiche

QUICHE   tart with egg and cream, meat or vegetable filling
QUICHE AGNÈS SOREL   quiche made with cream and cheese

QUICHE AU FROMAGE   cheese quiche
QUICHE DE CREVETTES   shrimp quiche
QUICHE FECOUSE   quiche with bacon, onions, cream
QUICHE FOUÉE   bacon and cream flan
QUICHE LORRAINE   egg and cheese pie
QUICHE RAMEQUIN FORESTIÈRE   thick sauce of eggs,
   cheese and mushrooms baked until brown

Rice

PILAF   rice cooked with onions and broth
PILAW   rice prepared with various other ingredients
POIVRON FARCI AU RIZ   pepper stuffed with rice
RISOTTO   rice braised in chicken stock with tomatoes and
   parmesan cheese
RISOTTO À LA PIÉMONTAISE   rice braised in chicken stock
RIZ   rice
RIZ À L'ÉTUVÉE AU BEURRE   steamed and buttered rice
RIZ À LA CRÉOLE   boiled rice with tomatoes and pimentos
RIZ AU LAIT   rice custard
RIZ COMPLET   brown rice
RIZ PILAF   rice boiled in a bouillon
RIZ SAUVAGE   wild rice
RIZ VALENCIENNE   rice, tomatoes, saffron, onions and
   shellfish
SALADE MADRAS   rice salad with tomatoes, green
   peppers, mustard, salad oil, wine vinegar, cooked rice
SALADE SHEPHERDESS   rice salad with hard boiled
   eggs, scallions, horseradish, sour cream
SOUBISE   puree of onions and rice

Salad Dressings

VINAIGRE   vinegar
VINAIGRETTE   French dressing for green salads, combination salads, and marinades

Salads

ALÉNOIS watercress

BARBE-DE-CAPUCIN wild endive

BATAVIA type of lettuce

CAPUCINE nasturtium used in salads like capers

CAROTTES RÂPÉES carrot salad with vinaigrette sauce

CHICORÉE curly endive

CHICORÉE AMÈRE bitter chicory

CHICORÉE FRISÉE curly leafed chicory

CHICORÉE SAUVAGE wild chicory

CHIFFONNADE DE CRABE crab, eggs, mayonnaise

COEUR DE PALMIER tender heart of palm

ENDIVE BELGE salad vegetable with crispy and bitter leaves

ESCAROLE green lettuce with slightly bitter taste

FEUILLE DE CHÊNE oak leaf lettuce

FRISÉE chicory

LAITUE lettuce

MACÉDOINE DE LÉGUMES salad of cooked vegetables in mayonnaise

MÂCHE lamb's lettuce, like a butter lettuce

MAYONNAISE dressing of egg yolks, vinegar or lemon juice

MESCLUN salad of mixed lettuces

NIÇOISE SALADE salad of vegetables, onions, anchovies, tunafish, artichokes and beans

POMMES DE TERRE À L'HUILE French potato salad, with vinegar, olive oil, herbs

ROMAINE romaine lettuce

SALADE salad

SALADE À LA BOUCHÈRE salad of boiled beef, potatoes and tomatoes

SALADE ALBIGNAC crayfish or chicken salad

SALADE ALLEMANDE salad of apple, herring and potato

SALADE ARLÉSIENNE salad of potatoes, artichokes, anchovies and tomatoes

SALADE CAUCHOISE   potato, celery and ham salad

SALADE CHIFFONNADE   shredded lettuce and sorrel in melted butter

SALADE COMPOSÉE   main course combination salad

SALADE D'ENDIVES   endive salad

SALADE D'ENDIVES ET DE BETTERAVES   endive and beet salad

SALADE DE BOEUF À LA PARISIENNE   beef and potato salad

SALADE DE CELÉRI   celery root in mustard mayonnaise dressing

SALADE DE CERVELAS   white sausage in vinaigrette sauce

SALADE DE COEURS D'ARTICHAUTS   artichoke hearts in oil and vinegar

SALADE DE CONCOMBRES   cucumber salad

SALADE DE FRUITS   fruit salad

SALADE DE HARENG   herring salad

SALADE DE LAITUE   lettuce salad

SALADE DE MOULES   mussel salad

SALADE DE MUSEAU DE BOEUF   marinated beef head-cheese salad

SALADE DE NOIX   nut and cheese salad

SALADE DE PISSENLITS AU LARD   dandelion leaves, bacon and new potatoes

SALADE DE POMMES DE TERRE   boiled potatoes, oil and vinegar dressing

SALADE DE QUEUES D'ÉCREVISSES   crayfish salad

SALADE DE RIZ À L'ORIENTALE   oriental rice salad

SALADE DE THON   tuna salad

SALADE DE TOMATES   tomato salad

SALADE DE VOLAILLE   chicken salad with mayonnaise

SALADE FLAMANDE   potato salad with salt herring

SALADE FOLLE   mixed salad, usually including green beans and liver

SALADE FRANCILLON   mussels and marinated potato salad

SALADE ITALIENNE   potatoes, asparagus tips, mayonnaise with anchovies, salami, olives, capers

SALADE JAPONAISE   tomato, orange and pineapple with sour cream

SALADE LYONNAISE   cooked diced vegetables, anchovies, oil and vinegar, onions, capers and hard eggs

SALADE MADRAS   rice salad with tomatoes, green peppers, mustard, salad oil, wine vinegar, cooked rice

SALADE MÊLÉE   mixed salad

SALADE MIMOSA   green salad with vinaigrette, sieved egg and herbs

SALADE NIÇOISE   salad with olives, anchovies and tuna fish

SALADE PANACHÉE   mixed salad

SALADE PAYSAN   quartered tomatoes, chopped onion, cucumbers, anchovies, oil and vinegar

SALADE PERNOLLET   truffle and crayfish salad

SALADE PORT ROYAL   apples, beans, potatoes, mayonnaise, hard boiled eggs

SALADE POTAGER   garden vegetable salad

SALADE RAPHAËL   lettuce, cucumber, asparagus, tomatoes, radishes and sauce

SALADE RUSSE   cooked vegetables in mayonnaise

SALADE SHEPHERDESS   rice salad with hard boiled eggs, scallions, horseradish, sour cream

SALADE TOURANGELLE   green bean and potato salad

SALADE VARIÉE   mixed salad

SALADE VERTE   green salad

SALADE VIGNERON   lettuce hearts with sour cream

SALADE WALDORF   apples, celery and walnuts in mayonnaise

SALADIER   salad bowl

SAUMON ROSE À LA PARISIENNE   cold poached salmon on mayonnaise and vegetables

TOTELOTS   hot noodle salad

Sauces

AIGRELETTE   tart sauce

AIL CRÉMAT   sauce made with garlic and olive oil for fish (Languedoc)

ALLEMANDE, SAUCE   cream sauce of egg yolks and lemon juice

ANCIENNE, À L'   cream sauce with mushrooms and wine

ARMENONVILLE   sauce of potatoes, tomatoes and artichokes

AURORE   tomato and cream sauce

BÉARNAISE   sauce of egg yolks, butter, shallots, tarragon, white wine, vinegar and herbs

BÉCHAMEL   white sauce with butter, flour, milk and onion

BERCY   meat stock with flour, butter and white wine

BEURRE BLANC   sauce of vinegar, shallots and butter

BEURRE NOIR   sauce of browned butter, lemon juice or vinegar

BEURRE VIERGE   butter sauce with salt, pepper and lemon juice

BIGARADE   orange sauce

BOLOGNAISE   sauce of tomatoes and vegetables, heavy garlic

BORDELAISE   brown sauce of shallots, red wine and bone marrow

BRETONNE   sauce of wine, carrots, leeks and celery

CÂPRES, SAUCE AUX   sauce from capers and butter

CARDINAL, SAUCE   sauce of pieces of lobster or crayfish

CHADEAU   a rich dessert type sauce

CHASSEUR, SAUCE   brown sauce with mushrooms, tomatoes, onions and white wine

CHIVRY, SAUCE   white wine sauce with herbs

CINGALAISE, À LA   curried

COLLIOURE, SAUCE   mayonnaise with anchovies and garlic

CRAPAUDINE, SAUCE   brown sauce made with onions, vinegar and spices

CRÈME AIGRE   sour cream

DEMI-GLACE   beef sauce lightened with consommé

DIABLE, SAUCE   sauce of vinegar, shallots and pepper

DUGLÈRE   tomato and herb sauce

ESPAGNOLE, SAUCE   vegetable, meat and tomato sauce

GASTRONOME, SAUCE   dark sauce made with white wine

GÉNOISE, SAUCE   sauce of nuts, cream and mayonnaise

GRAND VENEUR   a brown sauce with red currant jelly

INDIENNE, SAUCE À L'   with rice or curry

JOURNEAUX   chicken liver sauce

LIVORNAISE (SAUCE)   olive oil, egg yolks and anchovy paste

MARCHAND DE VIN   dark brown sauce made with meat and wine

MARGUERY, SAUCE   white wine and seafood sauce

MATELOTE SAUCE   sauce made with wine, garlic and shallots

MAYONNAISE   dressing of egg yolks, vinegar or lemon juice

MEURETTE   red wine sauce

MIRABEAU   anchovies, garlic, lemon juice

MONACO   with a green pea and caper sauce

MORNAY   thick, milk based sauce with flour, butter, egg yolks and cheese

MOUSSELINE SAUCE   Hollandaise sauce enriched with whipped cream

NESSELRODE   dessert or sauce containing fruits, chestnuts and whipped cream

NEWBURG, SAUCE   creamy sauce made with egg yolks, cream, sherry, and pieces of lobster

NORMANDE, SAUCE   fish cream sauce with mushrooms, wine or cider

PÉRIGUEUX, SAUCE DE   brown sauce with tomatoes, Madeira and truffles

PÉRIGOURDINE, SAUCE À LA   sauce of truffles and liver

PIQUANTE, SAUCE   spicy, brown sauce with small onions and pickles

POIVRADE, SAUCE   brown sauce dominated with black pepper

POULETTE, SAUCE   creamy white sauce made with egg yolks

PRINTANIÈRE, SAUCE   white sauce with green vegetables

PROVENÇALE, À LA sauce with garlic, tomatoes and olive oil

RAÏTO fish sauce of red wine, tomatoes, garlic and capers

RAVIGOTTE SAUCE cream sauce with shallots, herbs and spices

RIS DE VEAU À LA SUÉDOISE sweetbreads, tongue and horseradish sauce

ROBERT, SAUCE brown sauce made with onions, wine and vinegar

ROUENNAISE, SAUCE brown sauce containing ground duck livers

ROUILLE spicy sauce with olive oil, red peppers, tomatoes and garlic served with fish soups

ROUX butter and flour used as a thickener

SABAYON sweet sauce of egg yolks, sugar, wine and flavoring

SAUCE liquid dressing for food

SAUCE À LA CRESSONADE watercress sauce

SAUCE À LA DIABLE spicy sauce with white wine

SAUCE AIGRELETTE tart sauce

SAUCE AÏLLADA oil and garlic sauce

SAUCE ALBERT creamed horseradish sauce

SAUCE ALBERTINE sauce made with mushrooms and white wine

SAUCE ALLEMANDE cream sauce with egg yolks and lemon juice

SAUCE AMIRAL anchovy and herb sauce

SAUCE ANCIENNE cream sauce with mushrooms and wine

SAUCE ARMENONVILLE sauce of potatoes, tomatoes and artichokes

SAUCE AURORE creamy sauce with tomato puree

SAUCE AUX CÂPRES sauce made from fish concentrate, capers and butter

SAUCE AUX FRAISES fresh strawberry sauce

SAUCE AUX FRAMBOISES fresh raspberry sauce

SAUCE AUX RIS DE VEAU À LA SUÉDOISE sweetbreads, tongue and horseradish sauce

SAUCE BÉARNAISE   sauce of egg yolks, butter, shallots, tarragon, white wine, vinegar, herbs

SAUCE BÉCHAMEL   creamy white sauce with buttermilk

SAUCE BERCY   shallots, white wine in a creamy chicken sauce

SAUCE BIGARADE   orange sauce

SAUCE BOLOGNAISE   sauce of tomatoes and vegetables, heavy garlic

SAUCE BONNE FEMME   shallots, white wine, mushrooms and lemon juice

SAUCE BORDELAISE   brown sauce of shallots, red wine and bone marrow

SAUCE BRETONNE   creamy white sauce with strips of vegetables

SAUCE BRUNE   brown sauce from meat stock, onions and tomatoes

SAUCE CAFÉ DE PARIS   cream, mustard and herbs

SAUCE CARDINAL   sauce of cream with lobster pieces and herbs

SAUCE CHADEAU   sweet dessert sauce

SAUCE CHASSEUR   brown sauce with wine, mushrooms, onions

SAUCE CHIVRY   white wine sauce with herbs

SAUCE CHORON   tomato flavored bearnaise sauce

SAUCE COLLIOURE   anchovy and mayonnaise sauce

SAUCE CRAPAUDINE   brown sauce made with onions, vinegar and spices

SAUCE DEMI-GLACE   concentrated sauce lightened with consommé

SAUCE DIANE   peppery cream sauce

SAUCE DUGLÈRE   white sauce with shallots, white wine, tomatoes

SAUCE EN MEURETTE   red wine sauce

SAUCE ESPAGNOLE   vegetable, meat and tomato sauce

SAUCE FINANCIÈRE   cream, wine, spices, mushrooms, olives, truffles

SAUCE FORESTIÈRE   mushroom sauce

SAUCE GAILLARDE   hard egg yolks, oil, vinegar, capers, pickles

SAUCE GASTRONOME   dark sauce made with white wine

SAUCE GENEVOISE   sauce of fish stock, red wine and anchovy

SAUCE GÊNOISE   cold sauce of nuts, cream and mayonnaise

SAUCE GRAND VENEUR   pepper sauce with red currant jelly and cream

SAUCE GRIBICHE   hard boiled egg yolks with oil, vinegar, pickles

SAUCE HOLLANDAISE   sauce of egg yolks, butter and lemon juice

SAUCE HONGROISE   white sauce with onions and paprika

SAUCE INDIENNE   sauce with rice or curry

SAUCE ITALIENNE   brown sauce with mushrooms, ham and tarragon

SAUCE JOURNEAUX   chicken liver sauce

SAUCE LIVORNAISE   olive oil, egg yolks and anchovy paste

SAUCE MADÈRE   meat stock with Madeira wine

SAUCE MALTAISE   hollandaise sauce with grated orange peel

SAUCE MARCHAND DE VIN   dark brown sauce made with meat and wine

SAUCE MARGUERY   white wine and seafood sauce

SAUCE MATELOTE   fish sauce made with wine, anchovies and mushrooms

SAUCE MIRABEAU   anchovies, garlic, lemon juice

SAUCE MORNAY   creamy cheese sauce with eggs

SAUCE MOUSSELINE   hollandaise sauce with whipped cream

SAUCE MOUSSEUSE   butter with lemon juice and whipped cream

SAUCE NANTUA   white wine shrimp sauce with shrimp butter

SAUCE NAPOLITAINE   horseradish, red currant jelly and Madeira

SAUCE NESSELRODE   sauce containing fruits and chestnuts

SAUCE NIÇOISE   tomato and meat sauce

SAUCE NOISETTE   egg yolks and lemon in cream with butter added

SAUCE NORMANDE   fish cream sauce with mushrooms

SAUCE PARISIENNE   cream cheese, oil and lemon juice

SAUCE PAUVRE HOMME   stock, vinegar, shallots and breadcrumbs

SAUCE PÉRIGOURDINE   sauce with truffles and liver

SAUCE PÉRIGUEUX   brown sauce with tomatoes, Madeira wine and truffles

SAUCE PIBRONATA   spicy tomato and pepper sauce

SAUCE PIÉMONTAISE   onions, truffles, pine kernels and garlic

SAUCE PIQUANTE   spicy brown sauce with small onions and pickles

SAUCE POIVRADE   brown sauce dominated with pepper

SAUCE PORTUGAISE   tomato sauce with onions, garlic

SAUCE POULETTE   creamy white sauce with egg yolks

SAUCE PRINTANIÈRE   white sauce with green vegetables

SAUCE RAIFORT   horseradish sauce

SAUCE RAITO   fish sauce of red wine, tomatoes, garlic and walnuts

SAUCE RAVIGOTE   green herb sauce

SAUCE RÉMOULADE   mayonnaise, capers, mustard, anchovies

SAUCE RICHE   white sauce with lobster, butter and truffles

SAUCE ROBERT   sauce of white wine, onion and mustard

SAUCE ROUENNAISE   red wine sauce with liver

SAUCE ROUMAINE   spicy, sweet brown sauce with currants

SAUCE ROYALE   white chicken sauce

SAUCE RUSSE   white sauce with mustard, sugar and lemon juice

SAUCE SABAYON   sweet sauce of egg yolks, sugar, wine

SAUCE SAUPIQUET   spicy wine and vinegar sauce thickened with bread

SAUCE SMITANE   onion and heavy sour cream sauce

SAUCE SOUBISE   onion cream sauce
SAUCE ST. MALO   onions, mushrooms, mustard, anchovy
SAUCE SUPRÊME   thick chicken stock base
SAUCE TARTARE   mayonnaise, pickles, chives, capers and olives
SAUCE TOULONNAISE   onions, wine, pickle, capers and olives
SAUCE VALENCIENNE   tomato, rice, mushrooms, tongue and cheese
SAUCE VELOUTÉ   cream sauce usually made from chicken and vegetables
SAUCE VERTE   green sauce made from green vegetables with mayonnaise
SAUCE VINCENT   green herb mayonnaise sauce
SAUPIQUET   spicy wine and vinegar sauce thickened with bread
SMITANE   sauce of cream, onions, white wine and lemon juice
SOUBISE SAUCE   onion cream sauce
VALENCIENNE   tomato, rice, mushrooms, tongue and cheese
VELOUTÉ   a sauce, soup or dish having a smooth, creamy taste, also see Crème

Sausages

ALSACIENNE   with sauerkraut, ham and sausages
ANDOUILLE   chitterling sausage
ANDOUILLE DE VIRE   smoked pork and tripe sausage
ANDOUILLETTE   small chitterling sausage
ASSIETTE SALAMI   plate of various salamis
BOUDIN   sausage
BOUDIN BLANC   white sausage of veal, chicken or pork
BOUDIN DE VEAU   veal and bacon sausage
BOUDIN NOIR   pork blood sausage
BROCCANA   sausage-meat and veal pâté
CAPOUN   cabbage filled with rice and sausage

CAPOUN FASSUM   stuffed cabbage and sausage

CASSOULET PÉRIGOURDIN   stew of beans, mutton and sausage

CATALANE, SAUCISSE À LA   fried sausage with garlic

CERVELAS   sausage

CERVELAS EN BRIOCHE   pork sausage in brioche pastry

CHAMPENOISE (POTÉE)   stew of ham, sausage and cabbage

CHARCUTERIE ASSORTIE   assorted pork products

CHINONAISE   potatoes and sausage in cabbage

CHIPOLATAS   small pork sausages

CHORIZO   very spicy sausage

COPPA   a variety of sausage

COUDENAT   pork sausage

CRÉPINETTE   small spicy flat sausage

CRÉPINETTES TRUFFÉES   pork sausages with truffles

DIOT   pork sausage cooked in wine

DIOTS AU VIN BLANC   sausages cooked in white wine

ESTOUFFAT DE HARICOTS   stew of sausages or ham, white beans and pork

FARÇON   fried sausage and vegetable cake

FIGATELLI   spicy pork sausage

FRIAND ST. FLOUR   sausage meat in pastry

FROMAGE DE TÊTE   head cheese, usually pork

GAYETTES   sausage patties with pork liver and bacon

GRATIN DE POMMES DE TERRE SAUCISSON   sausage and potato casserole

HURE MARCASSIN   a head cheese prepared from boar

JÉSUS   sausage

JÉSUS DE MORTEAU   smoked sausage

KNACKWURST   sausage

LOUKINKA   garlic sausage

MORTADELLE   large sausage

OULADE   stew made from potatoes, cabbage, sausage and pork

RAGOÛT BIGOUDEN   stewed sausage with potato and onions

ROSETTE   large pork sausage served in slices
ROSETTE DE BOEUF   dried sausage
SABODET   sausage from pig's head
SALADE DE CERVELAS   white sausage in vinaigrette
   sauce
SALADE DE MUSEAU DE BOEUF   marinated beef head-
   cheese
SAUCE STUFFATU   meat sauce of tomatoes, onions and
   wine with pasta
SAUCISSE   small fresh sausage
SAUCISSE À LA CATALANE   sausage fried with garlic
SAUCISSE CHAUDE   warm sausage
SAUCISSE DE FRANCFORT   hot dog
SAUCISSE DE LYON   boiled coarse grained sausage
SAUCISSE DE STRASBOURG   red skinned hot dog
SAUCISSE DE TOULOUSE   mild country style pork sausage
SAUCISSE GRILLÉE   fried sausage
SAUCISSE PAYSANNE   country style sausage
SAUCISSE TIMBALE DE   sausage pâté in crust
SAUCISSON   large, dry salami like sausage
SAUCISSON À L'AIL   garlic sausage served warm
SAUCISSON CERVELAS   garlicky cured pork sausage
SAUCISSON CONFIT   duck, goose, pork cooked and
   preserved in its own fat
SAUCISSON COU D'OIE FARCI   neck skin of goose,
   stuffed with meat
SAUCISSON CRÉPINETTE   small sausage patty
SAUCISSON D'ARLES   dried, salami type sausage
SAUCISSON DE CAMPAGNE   country style sausage
SAUCISSON DE LYON   dried pork sausage with garlic,
   pepper and pork fat
SAUCISSON DE TOULOUSE   pork sausage, boiled then
   grilled
SAUCISSON EN BRIOCHE   sausage cooked in dough
SAUCISSON EN CROÛTE   sausage cooked in pastry crust
SAUCISSON SEC   dried sausage
SAUCISSONS VARIÉS   slices of mixed sausage

Seafood

ABLETTE   bleak, a freshwater fish
ACTINIE   sea anemone
AFRICAINE   with eggplant, mushrooms, potatoes and
   tomatoes
AIGLEFIN   fresh haddock
ALLEMANDE   with noodles and mashed potatoes
ALOSE   shad
ALOSE À LA CRÈME   shad in cream sauce
ALOSE ADOUR   herring stuffed and baked with ham
ALOSE AU FOUR   baked shad
ALOSE AVIGNONNAISE   fried shad, baked with sorrel
ALOSE LOIRE   shad broiled, then baked over sorrel
ALPHÉE   prawn-like shellfish
AMANDE DE MER   a small clam
ANCHOIS   anchovy
ANDALOUSE   with green peppers, eggplant and
   tomatoes
ANGES CHEVAL   grilled oysters with bacon
ANGUILLE   eel
ANGUILLE AU VERT   eel braised in green sauce
ANGUILLE FUMÉE   smoked eel
ANTIBOISE, À L'   with cheese, garlic, tomatoes and
   sardines or anchovy or tuna
ARAIGNÉE DE MER   spider crab
ARCACHON, HUÎTRE D'   oyster with a strong flavor
ARCHIDUC   with cream and paprika
ARIÉGEOISE   with cabbage, pork, potatoes, beans
ARLÉSIENNE   with eggplant, olives, onions, potatoes,
   rice and tomatoes
ASSIETTE DE FRUITS DE MER   seafood platter
ASSIETTE DE PÊCHEUR   assorted fish platter
ATHÉRINE   fried smelt
BADÈCHE   sea bass
BAR   bass
BAR DE MER   sea bass

BAR POCHÉ AU BEURRE BLANC   poached bass with
  white butter sauce
BAR RAYÉ   striped bass
BARBEAU   variety of carp
BARBUE   brill, a Mediterranean flatfish related to turbot
BARQUETTE ÉCOSSAISE   pastry shell with smoked salmon
BARQUETTE OSTENDAISE   pastry shells with creamed
  oysters
BASQUAISE   with ham and tomatoes or red peppers
BATELIÈRE   pastry shells with seafood filling
BAUDROIE   monkfish
BEIGNET DE POISSON   miniature fish balls
BEIGNET NIÇOIS   batter fried pieces of tunafish
BEIGNET SOUFFLÉ   fritter with fish or meat filling
BELON   oyster
BELONS, DEMI-DOUZAINE DE   a half dozen oysters
BELONS, DOUZAINE DE   a dozen oysters
BELUGA   caviar
BIGORNEAU   winkle, a small sea mollusk
BLANCHAILLE   whitebait fish, like a sprat
BLANCHAILLE FRITE   fried whitebait fish
BLANQUETTE   veal, lamb, chicken, seafood in white sauce
BOITELLE   cooked with mushrooms
BONITE   bonita, similar to tunafish
BOUFFI   smoked kipper
BOUILLITURE D'ANGUILLES   eels stewed in wine
BOULETTE   meatball or fishball
BOUQUET   large reddish shrimp
BOURRIDE   garlicky fish stew
BOURRIDE À L'AÏOLI   fish stew with garlic mayonnaise,
  from Provence
BRANDADE DE MORUE   creamed salt cod
BRÈME   bream; a carp fish
BROCHET   pike
BROCHET BADOISE   baked pike cooked with sour cream
BROCHETTE   meat or fish and vegetables on a skewer
BULOT   large sea snail

CABILLAUD   codfish

CABILLAUD AU FOUR   baked codfish

CABILLAUD BONNE FEMME   wine poached cod fish in creamy sauce

CAÏEU   giant mussel

CALAMAR   squid

CALMAR   squid

CANCALAISE   oysters and shrimps in cream wine sauce

CANNELON   puff-pastry with meat or fish filling

CAPELAN   codfish

CARAMOTE   large prawn

CARDINAL   garnish for fish, of mushrooms, truffles, scallops

CARDINAL, SAUCE   sauce of pieces of lobster or crayfish

CARDINALIZER   cooking shellfish in boiling salt water

CARPE   carp fish

CARPE AU JUIF   boiled carp served cold in aspic

CARPE POLONAISE   carp cooked in red wine with onions

CARRELET   flounder

CATALANE   eggplant, tomatoes, onions, peppers and rice

CATIGOT   eel stewed in wine and tomatoes

CAUDIÈRE   fish stew with mussels cooked with white wine

CAVIAR   sturgeon eggs

CAVIAR BLANC   mullet eggs

CAVIAR FRAIS   fresh fish eggs

CAVIAR MALOSSIL   fish eggs, lightly salted

CAVIAR NIÇOIS   anchovies, oil, fish eggs, usually served on toast

CÉVÉNOLE   with chestnuts and mushrooms

CHABLISIENNE   cooked and served in white wine

CHAUD-FROID DE SAUMON   cold salmon in a rich jellied sauce

CHAUDRÉE   seafood stew

CHAUDRÉE ROCHELAISE   fish stew of tiny fish and wine

CHAUSSON AUX MOULES   turnover stuffed with mussels

CHEVAINE OR CHEVESNE   type of carp

CHILIENNE   with rice and sweet peppers

CHIPIRON   small squid
CIVELLES FRITES   fried baby eels
CIVET DE LANGOUSTE   lobster stewed in wine, tomatoes and onions
CLOVISSE   clam
CLUPE   herring
COLIN   hake
COLIN À LA GRANVILLAISE   hake, like cod, served with shrimps
CONGRE   conger eel
COQUE   small clam like shellfish
COQUILLAGES   shellfish
COQUILLES-ST-JACQUES   scallops
COQUILLES-ST-JACQUES À LA MÉNAGÈRE   scallops sautéed with wine, onions, mushrooms
COQUILLES-ST-JACQUES AU GRATIN   scallops in wine with mushroom and tomato sauce
COQUILLES-ST-JACQUES BÉCHAMEL   scallops in shell with white sauce, browned
COQUILLES-ST-JACQUES CRÉOLE   scallops in wine with tomato fondue
COQUILLES-ST-JACQUES PARISIENNE   scallops and mushrooms in white wine sauce
COQUILLES-ST-JACQUES PROVENÇALE   scallops sautéed with garlic butter sauce, grated cheese, tomato, oven browned
CÔTES BLEUES   large oyster
COTRIADE   fish soup stew
COULIBIAC   fish in pastry baked then sliced
COULIBIAC DE SAUMON EN CROÛTE   salmon, rice and mushrooms baked in pastry
COURONNE DE RIZ AUX CREVETTES   creamed prawns in rice ring
COURQUIGNOISE   fish stew in white wine with mussels
CRABE   crab
CRABE À LA PARISIENNE   crab with mayonnaise and chopped vegetables

CRABE À LA RUSSE   crab in the shell with mayonnaise and capers

CRAPAUD   toad

CRAQUELOT   smoked, salted herring

CRÉOLE   with rice, sweet peppers and tomatoes

CRÊPES ROULÉES FARCIES   crepes with creamed shellfish, gratinéed in wine and cheese sauce

CREUSE   elongated, crinkle shelled oyster

CREVETTE   shrimp

CREVETTE EN BROCHETTE   shrimps broiled on skewer

CREVETTE GRISE   small shrimp that turns gray when cooked

CREVETTE ROSE   small shrimp that turns red when cooked

CRISTE MARINE   edible algae growing on rock

CROQUE AU SEL   raw, with salt

CROQUETTE   ground meat, fish, fowl or vegetables, coated in breadcrumbs and deep fried

CROUSTADE DE CREVETTES NANTUA   pastry with shrimp in wine sauce

CROUSTADE DE FRUITS DE MER   pastry filled with seafood

CROUSTADE DE LANGOUSTES   pastry shell with lobster in cream sauce

CROÛTE   in pastry

CRUSTACÉ   shellfish

CUISSES DE GRENOUILLE   frogs' legs

DARD   freshwater carp

DARNE   slice of fish

DARNE DE SAUMON GRILLÉE   grilled salmon steak

DARNE DE SAUMON GRILLÉE AU BEURRE D'ESCARGOT   broiled salmon steak with garlic and herb butter

DARNE MONTMORENCY   salmon, mushrooms and olives

DAURADE   sea bream

DEAUVILLAISE, SOLE À LA   poached sole with onions and cream

DEMOISELLE DE CHERBOURG   small lobster

DIABLE   very spicy, peppery sauce

DIABLE DE MER   monkfish

DIEPPOISE, À LA   wine, mussels, shrimp, mushrooms and cream

DORADE   bream

DOS   back

ÉCREVISSE   freshwater crayfish

ÉCREVISSE À LA NAGE   crayfish simmered in white wine, vegetables and herbs

ÉCREVISSES À LA LIÉGEOISE   crayfish with butter sauce

ÉGLEFIN   haddock

ENCORNET   small squid

ÉPERLAN   smelt, fish like a large sardine

ESPADON   swordfish

ESQUINADO   spider crab

ESTOFINADO   fish stew with dried cod cooked in walnut oil with eggs, garlic and cream

ESTURGEON   sturgeon

ÉTRILLE   small crab

FAVOUILLE   small crab

FÉRA   salmon type of lake fish

FILETS D'ANCHOIS   fillets of anchovies

FILETS DE POISSON MORNAY   fish fillets gratinéed with cheese

FILETS DE POISSON, SOUFFLÉ DE   fish soufflé on a platter

FILETS DE POISSONS GRATINÉS AU FOUR   fish fillets baked with cheese

FILETS DE POISSONS POCHÉS AU VIN BLANC   fish poached in wine

FILETS DE SOLE AMANDINE   fillets of sole cooked with butter and almonds

FILETS DE SOLE BONNE FEMME   sole with mushroom and wine sauce

FILETS DE SOLE CALYPSO   sole rolled up with finely ground lobster

FILETS DE SOLE FRITS   fried fillet of sole
FILETS DE SOLE SYLVESTRE   fish poached in wine with
   vegetables
FINE CLAIRE   oyster that is specially fattened
FINES CLAIRES   oysters that have been fattened up
FLET   flounder
FLÉTAN   halibut
FREMIS   lightly cooked oysters
FRETINS   fried sardines
FRIAND À LA MARSEILLAISE   pastry shell filled with
   tunafish
FRICASSÉE   meat, poultry or fish braised in wine or
   butter with cream
FRICASSÉE DE VOLAILLE ET D'ÉCREVISSES   chicken
   and crayfish stewed in cream and wine
FRITURE DE LA LOIRE   small deep-fried fish, like sardines
FRUITS DE MER   seafood
FUMÉES, MOULES   smoked mussels
FUMET   fish stock
GAMBAS   large prawns
GARDON   variety of carp
GEBIE   small shellfish
GOUJON   sardine-like freshwater fish
GRATIN (AU)   dish with a browned cheese and crusty
   breadcrumb topping over cream sauce
GRATIN DE FRUITS DE MER   shellfish
GRATIN DE QUEUES D'ÉCREVISSES   crayfish
GRENOUILLE   frog
GRENOUILLE BRESSANE   frog's legs in cream sauce
GRENOUILLE, CUISSES DE   frog's legs
GRENOUILLE PROVENÇALE   fried frogs' legs
GRILLADE AU FENOUIL   grilled with fennel, usually fish
GRONDIN   ocean fish used in stews and bouillabaisse
GRYPHÉE   Portuguese oyster
GUITARE   sea skate
GYMNÈTRE   Mediterranean codfish
HACHIS   minced or chopped meat or fish, like hash

HARENG   herring
HARENG BLANC   salt herring
HARENG FRAIS   fresh herring
HARENG FUMÉ   smoked herring
HARENG LUCAS   smoked herring in mustard mayonnaise sauce
HARENG ROULÉ   marinated herring
HARENG SALÉ   salted kippered herring
HARENG SAUR   red herring
HÉNON   cockle, like small sea clam
HOMARD   lobster
HOMARD À L'AMÉRICAINE   lobster pieces sautéed in butter, flamed with cognac, then simmered in wine and vegetables
HOMARD À LA CHARENTAISE   lobster in cream sauce with cognac and grape juice
HOMARD À LA CRÈME   lobster with cream sauce
HOMARD À LA PARISIENNE   lobster pieces served with mixed vegetables in the shell
HOMARD À LA SUÉDOISE   baked lobster meat, anchovies and cream sauce
HOMARD CALVAISE   lobster in spicy tomato sauce
HOMARD CARDINAL   lobster flamed in brandy
HOMARD GRATINÉ FROMAGE   lobster steamed in wine and gratineed
HOMARD NEWBURG   lobster sautéed in Madeira wine and cream sauce
HOMARD THERMIDOR   lobster simmered in wine, butter, mushrooms; flamed and gratinéed with cheese
HUÎTRE   oyster
HUÎTRE DE BELON   flat, pinkish oyster
HUÎTRE FINE CLAIRE   like bluepoint oyster
HUÎTRE PORTUGAISE   small oyster
HURE DE SAUMON   pâté prepared with salmon
KIPPER   smoked herring
LAITANCE   fish roe milt, fish eggs
LAMPROIE   lamprey, an eel-shaped fish

LAMPROIE À LA BORDELAISE   eel in red wine
LANGOUSTE   lobster
LANGOUSTE À LA DIABLE   spicy baked lobster
LANGOUSTE SÉTOISE   lobster in spicy tomato sauce
  with brandy
LANGOUSTE WINTERTHUR   lobster with shrimp and
  mushroom, gratinéed
LANGOUSTINE   large prawn
LAVARET   fish related to the salmon
LIÉGEOISE   made with juniper berries and gin
LIEU JAUNE   pollack, a small saltwater fish
LIMANDE   fish similar to sole
LIMANDE SOLE   lemon sole
LINGUE   cod fish
LISETTE   small mackerel
LORRAINE, À LA   braised in wine
LOTTE   monkfish
LOUBINE   gray mullet fish
LOUP   bass fish
LOUP AU FENOUIL   sea bass flambéed in brandy
LOUP DE MER   Mediterranean fish, similar to striped bass
LYONNAISE, À LA   garnished with onions; in the style of
  Lyons
MAQUEREAU   mackerel
MAQUEREAU À LA BOULONNAISE   poached mackerel
  with mussels
MAQUEREAU AU VIN BLANC   mackerel poached in
  white wine
MAQUEREAU EN PAPILLOTE   mackerel baked in paper
MAQUEREAU GRILLÉ   grilled mackerel
MAQUEREAU MARINÉ   pickled or marinated mackerel
MARENNES   flat shelled, green tinged plate oysters
MARINÉ   marinated
MARINIÈRE   seafood in white wine and spices
MARINIÈRE, MOULES   mussels in white wine with
  onions, shallots, butter and herbs
MARMITE DIEPPOISE   fish stewed in white wine and cream

MATELOTE   fish stew
MATELOTE CANOTIÈRE   carp and eel stew
MATELOTE D'ANGUILLE   eel and fish stew
MAYONNAISE, POISSON À LA   fish with mayonnaise
MERLAN   whiting
MERLU   dried codfish
MERLUCHE   dried codfish
MEUNIÈRE   fish seasoned, floured, fried in butter
MORUE   salted or dried codfish
MORUE AUX ÉPINARDS   codfish prepared with spinach
MORUE PROVENÇALE   salt cod with garlic and onion
   sauce
MORUE SALÉE   salt cod
MOSTELE   small Mediterranean fish
MOUCLADE   creamy mussel stew with curry
MOULE   mussel
MOULE D'ESPAGNE   large raw mussels
MOULE FARCIE   stuffed mussel
MOULE NORMANDE   mussel in wine and cream sauce
MOULES MARINIÈRE   boiled mussels in white wine
   with shallots and parsley
MOUSSE   beaten egg whites or whipped cream; meat,
   poultry or fish finely ground and served in a mold
MOUSSELINE   ground fish beaten with egg white and
   cream, cooked in patties
MOUSSELINE DE POISSON MARÉCHALE   fish cakes
   with vinegar and wine, butter and shallot sauce
MULET   grey mullet fish
MYE   clam
NAGE, À LA   cooked and served in bouillon poaching
   liquid
NEWBURG   lobster prepared with Madeira, egg yolks
   and cream
NIÇOISE, À LA   refers to dishes with onions, garlic, olive
   oil, tomatoes, anchovies
NORMANDE, À LA   fish or meat cooked with apple
   cider; apple dessert with cream

OEUF DE POISSON   egg with fish roe

OIE   goose

OMBLE   lake trout, like salmon

OMBLE-CHEVALIER   felchen from Lake Constance

OURSIN   sea urchin

PACARET   made with sherry

PAGRE   pompano type fish in bream family

PAIN DE BROCHET D'ANGOULÊME   fish loaf of pike

PAIN DE POISSON   loaf of ground fish

PALOURDE   medium size clam

PANÉ   prepared with breadcrumbs

PAPILLOTE, EN   cooked in parchment paper or foil envelope

PÂTÉ CHAUD AU SAUMON   salmon pie

PAUCHOUSE   fresh water fish stew

PAUPIETTE   slice of chicken, fish or meat filled with
   another mixture, rolled up and sautéed

PERCE-PIERRE   edible algae growing on rock

PERCHE   lake fish

PETIT GRATIN DE CRABE AU VIN BLANC   crab meat
   in white wine sauce baked with cheese

PETITES BOUCHÉES   small pastry shells filled with fish
   or other ingredients

PÉTONCLE   tiny scallop

PÉTONCLE RAGOÛT DE   scallop stew

PIBALLES   small eels

PIEUVRE   octopus

PILCHARD   sardine

PISSALADIÈRE   Provençale onion and anchovy pie

PLATEAU DE FRUITS DE MER   seafood platter with raw
   and cooked shellfish, including oysters, clams, mussels,
   crabs

PLIE   fish like sole or flounder

PLOUSE   codfish

POCHÉ   poached

POCHOUSE   freshwater fish stew prepared with white wine

POCHOUSE BOURGUIGNONNE   with eel and other fish
   in wine

POISSON   fish
POISSON À LA PROVENÇALE   white fish fried with onions, garlic, tomatoes, fresh herbs
POISSON BASQUE   fish sautéed in clam juice, white wine, mashed tomatoes, scallions
POISSON COCOTTE   swordfish or tuna simmered in a skillet with onions, butter and white wine
POISSON CÔTE AZUR   fish simmered with tomatoes, fennel, thyme, garlic, peppercorns and wine
POISSON D'EAU DOUCE   freshwater fish
POISSON DE LAC   lake fish
POISSON DE MER   saltwater fish
POISSON DE RIVIÈRE   river fish
POISSON DU HAVRE, FILETS DE   fish sautéed then flamed with whiskey, clam juice, heavy cream, lemon juice
POISSON FARCI À LA FLORENTINE   baked fish with spinach stuffing
POISSON MAÎTRE D'HÔTEL   fish boiled in saucepan with thin slices of lemon
POISSON MEUNIÈRE   fish sautéed with flour, butter, lemon juice
POISSON ORLY   fish fillets deep fried in batter with tomato sauce
POISSON POCHÉ AU COURT BOUILLON   fish poached in fish stock
PORTUGAISES   elongated, crinkle-shell oysters
POT-AU-FEU D'HOMARD   lobster and seafood stew
POULPE   octopus
POUTARGUE   paste of mullet roe
POUTINA NONNAT   very small fried fish
PRAIRE   small clam
QUENELLE   dumpling, usually of veal, fish or poultry
QUENELLE DE BROCHET   dumpling of ground pike
QUENELLE DE POISSON   puree of fish formed into balls and poached
QUEUE D'ÉCRIVISSES   crayfish tails

QUICHE   tart with egg and cream, meat or vegetable filling

QUIMPER   mackerel

RAIE   skate-like fish

RAIE AU BEURRE NOIR   skate with black butter

RASCASSE   Mediterranean fish used for soup and stews

ROCHES   large Portuguese oyster

ROUGET   red Mediterranean fish

ROUGET AU FENOUIL   rouget cooked with olive oil, bacon and fennel

ROUGET MEUNIÈRE   red mullet fried in butter

ROYAN   pilchard, similar to herring or sardine

SAINT-PIERRE   sea fish

SALADE DE MOULES À LA PROVENÇALE   mussel salad with chopped onion fried in olive oil with tomatoes and garlic

SALMIS DE POISSONS   mixed seafood stew with wine

SALPICON   diced vegetables, meat and/or fish in a sauce

SANDRE   perchlike freshwater fish

SARDINE   small fish

SARDINE À L'HUILE   sardine in olive oil

SARDINE NIÇOISE   boneless sardine cooked in white wine, mushrooms and spices

SARDINES AUX OEUFS AU CITRON   sardines with hard boiled eggs and lemon

SAUMON   salmon

SAUMON ALSATIEN   boiled in wine and onions over creamed spinach

SAUMON D'ÉCOSSE   Scottish salmon

SAUMON DE NORVÈGE   cold salmon slices in aspic

SAUMON DU RHIN   Rhine salmon

SAUMON FUMÉ   smoked salmon

SAUMON GLACÉ   cold salmon in aspic jelly

SAUMON POCHÉ   poached whole salmon

SAUTERELLE   shrimp

SCAMPI   shellfish similar to shrimp prepared with garlic

SEICHE   large squid or cuttlefish

SOLE   flat flounder-like fish

SOLE ARLÉSIENNE   sole cooked with garlic, tomatoes and onions

SOLE AU GRATIN   baked sole with shallots, mushrooms and breadcrumbs

SOLE AU VIN BLANC   sole cooked in cream, egg yolks and white wine

SOLE CHAUCHAT   poached sole in Mornay sauce with fried potatoes

SOLE COLBERT   fillets of sole, covered with breadcrumbs and fried

SOLE CUBAT   poached sole with pureed mushrooms in cream sauce

SOLE INDIENNE   sole with tomatoes, coconut milk, cream and curry powder

SOLE MARGUERY   sole, shrimps and mushrooms with a cream sauce

SOLE MÉNAGÈRE   sole baked on vegetables with red wine

SOLE MURAT   sole fried with potatoes and artichoke

SOLE NORMANDE   sole poached in wine in cream sauce with oysters, crayfish

SOLE OLGA   poached sole stuffed into baked potatoes with a covering of shrimp sauce

SOLE SYLVETTE   sole sautéed with vegetables and sherry

ST-PIERRE   mild, flat, white ocean fish

STOCAFICADA   dried salt cod stewed in oil with vegetables

SUPRÊME   boneless breast of poultry or a fillet of fish

TACAUD   type of codfish

TANCHE   variety of carp

TERRINE   earthenware container for baking meat, game, fish or vegetable mixture

TERRINE D'ANGUILLE   eel cooked in an earthenware container

TERRINE DE BROCHET   finely ground pike, usually served as an appetizer

THON   tuna

TIORO   fish stew with tomato, onion and garlic

TOMATE À L'ANTIBOISE   marinated tomato stuffed with tuna

TRANCHE DE CABILLAUD   codfish steaks

TRUITE   trout

TRUITE AMANDINE   trout served with slivers of toasted almonds

TRUITE ARC-EN CIEL   rainbow trout

TRUITE AU BLEU   trout poached in vinegar bouillion

TRUITE DE LAC   lake trout

TRUITE DE RIVIÈRE   river trout

TRUITE GOURMET   trout with mayonnaise and artichokes

TRUITE MONTBARDOISE   trout stuffed with spinach

TRUITE MONTGOLFIER   boneless trout, white wine and lobster sauce

TRUITE SAUMONÉE   salmon trout

TRUITE SAUMONÉE EN GELÉE   cold salmon trout in aspic

TRUITE VIVANTE   trout alive till immediately before cooking

TRUITES AUX AMANDES   trout with almonds

TURBOT   flat sea fish like flounder

TURBOT AU CHAMPAGNE   poached in white wine or champagne

TURBOTIN   turbot

VANGEREN   type of carp

VAUCLUSIENNE   fried in olive oil, served with lemon juice

VAUDOISE   variety of carp

VÉNUS   sea cockle, a shellfish

WATERZOOI   chicken or fish stew in creamy sauce

ZINGARA   with tomato, ham and mushrooms

Soufflés

FILETS DE POISSON, SOUFFLÉ DE   fish soufflé on a platter

OEUF POCHÉ SOUFFLÉ À LA FLORENTINE   soufflé of poached egg on creamed spinach

OMELETTE SOUFFLÉ À LA LIQUEUR   liqueur flavored soufflé

RAMEQUIN FORESTIÈRE   thick sauce of eggs, cheese and mushrooms baked until brown

SOUFFLÉ   light, sweet or piquant mixture served either hot or cold, containing whipped egg whites to puff up when baked

SOUFFLÉ À L'ORANGE, FLAMBÉ   rum, orange and macaroon soufflé, flamed

SOUFFLÉ AU CHOCOLAT   chocolate soufflé

SOUFFLÉ AU FROMAGE   cheese soufflé in ramekins

SOUFFLÉ AU FROMAGE OEUFS MOLLETS   cheese soufflé with boiled eggs

SOUFFLÉ AU HOMARD   lobster soufflé

SOUFFLÉ AUX FRAMBOISES   raspberry soufflé

SOUFFLÉ AUX FRUITS   soufflé made with fruit preserves or pieces of fruit

SOUFFLÉ DE LÉGUMES   puree of cooked vegetables

SOUFFLÉ GRAND MARNIER   orange liqueur soufflé

SOUFFLÉ MOUSSELINE   cheese soufflé made with cream

SOUFFLÉ NORMAND   soufflé with calvados and apples

SOUFFLÉ OMELETTE   puffy omelet

SOUFFLÉ PALMYRE   soufflé made with macaroons or cake crumbs

SOUFFLÉ ROTHSCHILD   vanilla soufflé with fruit

Soup

AIGO BOUIDO   garlic soup over bread, sprinkled with cheese

AIGO SAU   fish soup with potatoes, garlic, tomato, parsley, onion, bay leaf

AIL, SOUPE À   garlic and milk soup, served with cheese

ARGENTEUIL, CRÈME   asparagus soup

ASIMINU   fish soup

ASSIETTE CREUSE   soup plate

BAGRATION, SOUPE   veal or fish soup with macaroni

BALVET   soup of pureed peas

BIJANE   cold wine and bread soup
BISQUE   shellfish soup
BISQUE D'ÉCREVISSES   crayfish soup
BISQUE DE CREVETTES   shrimp bisque
BISQUE DE HOMARD   lobster chowder
BONNE FEMME, POTAGE   potato, carrot and leek soup
BORSCHT   beet soup, Russian style
BOUILLABAISSE   fish stew soup
BOUILLABAISSE AUX ÉPINARDS   spinach soup with
   potatoes, served on bread with poached eggs
BOUILLABAISSE MARSEILLAISE   Mediterranean fish
   chowder with onions, leeks, olive oil, tomatoes, garlic
BOUILLON   a light soup or broth (also see consommé)
BOURGUIGNON, POTAGE   heavy vegetable soup with
   sausage and pork
BOURRIDE   garlicky fish stew
BRAOU BOUFFAT   soup of rice and cabbage
BROU   soup made from cabbage and rice
BRUXELLOIS, POTAGE   Brussels sprout soup
CANCALAIS   fish consommé
CATALANE, SOUPE   tomato and onion soup
CÉLESTINE, POTAGE   soup of leeks and potatoes
CÈPES, POTAGE DE   dried mushroom soup
CHABRILLAN   puree of tomato soup
CHAMONIX   ground chicken, hard egg in chicken broth
   with cream
CHAMPIGNONS, POTAGE AUX   mushroom soup
CONCOMBRE, POTAGE DE   cream of cucumber soup,
   hot or cold
CONDÉ, POTAGE   mashed red bean soup
CONSOMMÉ   clear soup
CONSOMMÉ À L'ALLEMANDE   double strength beef
   soup with frankfurter slices
CONSOMMÉ À L'ALSACIENNE   clear beef soup with
   noodles
CONSOMMÉ À L'AMÉRICAINE   double strength beef
   soup with green peas

CONSOMMÉ À L'IRLANDAISE   clear soup with mutton, barley and vegetables

CONSOMMÉ À L'OEUF   clear soup with a raw egg

CONSOMMÉ À LA BOUCHÈRE   clear beef soup with bone-marrow and cabbage

CONSOMMÉ À LA GAULOISE   chicken consommé with cockscombs and kidneys

CONSOMMÉ À LA PARISIENNE   chicken consommé with vegetables

CONSOMMÉ À LA REINE   thickened chicken consommé with strips of chicken

CONSOMMÉ ADÈLE   clear soup with vegetables

CONSOMMÉ ALEXANDRA   clear chicken soup with chicken balls and lettuce

CONSOMMÉ AUX CHEVEUX D'ANGE   clear soup with thin noodles

CONSOMMÉ AUX VERMICELLES   clear soup with thin noodles

CONSOMMÉ BLANC   strained soup from veal and vegetables

CONSOMMÉ CANCALAISE   fish consommé with pike, oysters and parsley

CONSOMMÉ CARDINAL   clear fish soup with lobster balls

CONSOMMÉ CÉLESTINE   clear soup with chicken and noodles or crêpes

CONSOMMÉ COLBERT   clear soup with poached eggs, spring vegetables

CONSOMMÉ COMMODORE   fish consommé with clams and tomatoes

CONSOMMÉ CROÛTES AU POT   beef soup, vegetables and croutons

CONSOMMÉ DE GIBIER   game soup

CONSOMMÉ DE LÉGUMES   clear soup containing vegetables

CONSOMMÉ DE POULE   chicken broth

CONSOMMÉ DE TORTUE   turtle consommé with Madeira and turtle pieces

CONSOMMÉ DE TORTUE CLAIR   turtle soup with turtle meat and sherry

CONSOMMÉ DE VOLAILLE   broth from chicken, turkey, goose, duck

CONSOMMÉ DOUBLE   double strength broth

CONSOMMÉ EN GELÉE   jellied consommé

CONSOMMÉ FLIP   consommé of leeks and ham

CONSOMMÉ JOCKEY CLUB   clear chicken soup

CONSOMMÉ JULIENNE   clear soup with shredded vegetables

CONSOMMÉ MADRILÈNE   consommé with fresh tomato and herbs

CONSOMMÉ MERCÉDÈS   chicken consommé with sherry, sliced cock's kidneys

CONSOMMÉ MONACO   chicken consommé with cheese flavored rounds

CONSOMMÉ NEMROD   game consommé with port

CONSOMMÉ ORLÉANS   chicken consommé, cream, tomato puree and pistachios

CONSOMMÉ PORTO   clear soup with port wine

CONSOMMÉ PRINCESSE   clear soup with chicken and asparagus tips

COTRIADE   fish soup stew

COURT-BOUILLON   broth, or aromatic poaching liquid

COUSINETTE   sour soup of sorrel, spinach, chicory and Swiss chard

CRÉCY   carrot soup

CRÈME AUX POIREAUX   cream of leek soup

CRÈME D'ASPERGES   cream of asparagus soup

CRÈME D'ÉPINARDS   cream of spinach soup

CRÈME DE BOLETS   cream of boletus mushroom soup

CRÈME DE CÉLERI   cream of celery soup

CRÈME DE CHAMPIGNONS   cream of mushroom soup

CRÈME DE CRESSON   cream of watercress soup

CRÈME DE LAITUE   cream of lettuce soup

CRÈME DE LÉGUMES   cream of vegetable soup

CRÈME DE POULET   cream of chicken soup

CRÈME DE TOMATES   cream of tomato soup
CRÈME DE VOLAILLE   cream of chicken soup
CRÈME ÉVITA   cold soup made with tomatoes and cream
CRÈME VICHYSSOISE   cold potato and leek soup; very
   creamy
CRÈME VICHYSSOISE GLACÉE   iced potato and leek soup
CRESSON, POTAGE DE   watercress soup
CRESSON, POTAGE AU   watercress soup
CROÛTES AU POT   cheese and bread soup
CULTIVATEUR, SOUPE   soup made with vegetables,
   pork and potatoes
DARBLAY   cream of potato soup
DIABLOTIN   cheese croutons served with soup
DU BARRY, POTAGE   cream of cauliflower soup
ÉCHALOTES, POTAGE AUX   onion soup made with
   shallots
ELZEKARIA   bean and cabbage soup
ÉSAÜ   thick lentil soup
FARCIDURE   vegetable soup dumpling
FERMIÈRE, POTAGE À LA   soup of shredded vegetables
   and beans
FLORENTINE, POTAGE   cream of spinach soup
FOIE DE VOLAILLE, POTAGE DE   cream of chicken liver
   soup
FONDS DE CUISINE   homemade beef and chicken stocks
FONTANGES   soup of peas with cream
FRICADELLES   chopped meat patties, may have onion
   and potato, added to soups
GARBURE   soup of cabbage, carrots, beans and salt pork
GENTILHOMME   pureed lentil soup
GERMINY, POTAGE   sorrel and chicken soup
GRATINÉE   soup with cheese and croutons browned in
   the oven to melt cheese
GRATINÉE LYONNAISE   beef consommé
GRATINÉE, SOUPE   onion soup
GRENOUILLE, POTAGE DE   frogs' leg soup
IMPÉRIAL   cream of celery soup

INDIENNE, POTAGE À L'   cream soup with chicken, rice and curry

JUBILÉ, POTAGE   pea soup with vegetables

JULIENNE, BOUILLON   bouillon with vegetables

JULIENNE, POTAGE   vegetable soup

LAMBALLE   soup of pureed peas thickened with tapioca

LÉGUMES, POTAGE DE   vegetable soup

LENTILLE (POTAGE DE)   lentil soup

LONGCHAMP   peas, sorrel and chervil soup

LONGUEVILLE   soup with leeks and peas

MAGISTÈRE   meat and vegetable soup

MARIGNY   pea soup with French beans and peas

MARMITE   a rich meat soup

MAYORQUINA   cabbage and tomato soup with onions and leeks

MEHLSUPPE   leek and onion soup

MIJOT   soup of red wine and bread

MILANAISE, À LA   vegetable, ham and sausage soup with grated cheese

MIQUE SARLADAISE   soup with dumpling made with corn flour and pork fat

MONGLE   pea and tomato soup

MONTAGNARDE   vegetable soup with grated cheese

MOURTAYROL   ham, chicken, beef, and vegetable soup

MULLIGATAWNY   curry soup with onions and potatoes

NOUZILLARDS AU LAIT   chestnut and milk soup

OUILAT   onion soup with beans, leeks and cheese

OUILLADE   soup of cabbage and beans

PARMENTIER, POTAGE   potato soup

PETITE MARMITE   clear, strong bouillon with meat, vegetables, grated cheese, served in earthenware pots

PIROGUIS   unsweetened pastry filled with meat or cheese, usually served hot with soup

PISTOU, SOUPE AU   garlic and vegetable soup with thin pasta

PORTUGAISE   thick soup with pimentos and tomatoes

POT-AU-FEU   broth in which meat and vegetables are cooked

POTAGE   soup, also see potée, consommé
POTAGE À LA REINE   cream of chicken soup
POTAGE AU VERMICELLE   noodle soup
POTAGE AUX LENTILLES   lentil soup
POTAGE DE VOLAILLE   chicken broth
POTAGE DU JOUR   soup of the day
POTAGE HONGROIS   goulash soup
POTAGE OXTAIL   oxtail soup
POTAGE PORTUGAIS   tomato soup
POTAGE ST. CLOUD   thick soup of pureed peas with croutons
POTAGE ST. GERMAIN   pea soup
POTÉE   thick stewlike soup
POTÉE COMTOISE   soup of cabbage, potato and sausage
POULE AU POT   chicken in the pot, chicken soup
PURÉE BRETONNE   pureed bean soup
PURÉE DE POIS CASSÉS   split pea soup
QUEUE DE BOEUF, POTAGE DE   oxtail soup
SALDA   soup of bacon, sausage, cabbage and beans
SANTE   leek, potato and vegetable soup
SAVOYARDE   vegetable soup with grated cheese
SOBRONADE   thick soup of pork, white beans, turnips
   and onions
SOISSONNAISE, SOUPE   haricot bean soup
SOLFERINO   thick soup of pureed tomatoes, leeks and
   potatoes
SOUPE   peasant style soup, also see consommé, poteé and
   potage
SOUPE À L'AIL   garlic soup
SOUPE À L'OIGNON   onion soup
SOUPE À L'OIGNON GRATINÉE   onion soup gratinéed
   with cheese
SOUPE À L'OIGNON, MAISON   homemade French
   onion soup
SOUPE À L'OSEILLE   sorrel soup
SOUPE À LA BIÈRE   beer and onion soup
SOUPE AU PISTOU   vegetable soup with garlic, basil and
   cheese

SOUPE AUX CERISES   hot cherry soup

SOUPE AUX CHOUX   cabbage soup

SOUPE AUX CUISSES DE GRENOUILLES   frogs' legs soup

SOUPE AUX LÉGUMES   vegetable soup

SOUPE AUX MOULES   cream of mussel soup

SOUPE BERGER   onion and garlic soup

SOUPE DE POISSONS   soup of pureed fish with hot chili and garlic

SOUPE DE POULET   chicken soup

SOUPE DU JOUR   soup of the day

SOUPE ÉPAUTRE   soup stew with meat, vegetables and garlic

SOUPE MONTAGNARDE   thick vegetable soup with cheese

SOUPE ORLÉANAISE   potato soup flavored with green herbs

SOUPE PÊCHEUR   fish soup

SOUPE REINE   chicken soup with rice

SOUPE VENDANGES   country soup of meat and vegetables

THOURIN POTAGE   milk-onion soup with cheese on bread

TORTUE VÉRITABLE, SOUPE DE   real turtle soup

TOULIA   onion soup with tomatoes, leeks, cheese and garlic

VELOUTÉ   a sauce, soup or dish having a smooth, creamy taste, also see Crème

VELOUTÉ D'OIGNON   cream of onion soup

VELOUTÉ DE TOMATE   cream of tomato soup

VELOUTÉ DE VOLAILLE   cream of chicken soup

VELOUTÉ DE VOLAILLE LA SÉNÉGALAISE   curried turkey soup, hot or cold

VICHYSSOISE   chilled, pureed, leek and potato soup

VICHYSSOISE À LA RUSSE   cold leek and potato soup with beets and sour cream

XAVIER   creamy rice soup

ZIMINU   fish soup

Spices

ANETH   dill
ANETH DOUX   fennel
ANIS   anise
AROMATES   spices and herbs
BAIES ROSES   pink peppercorns
BARBOTINE   aromatic herb
BASILIC   basil
BOUQUET GARNI   bag of herbs cooked in stew or soup
CANNELLE   cinnamon
CARI   curry
CARVI   caraway seeds
CAYENNE   hot red pepper
CERFEUIL   chervil
CLOU DE GIROFLE   clove
CORIANDRE   coriander, either fresh herbs or dried seeds
CUMIN   caraway, cumin
CURCUMA   turmeric
DIJON   type of mustard
DIJONNAISE   made with mustard
ÉPICE   spice
ESTRAGON   tarragon
FENOUIL   fennel
FINES HERBES   mixture of herbs; parsley, chives, tarragon
FRITURE   oil used for deep frying or fried fish
GERMINY   garnish of sorrel
GINGEMBRE   ginger
GIROFLE   cloves
GRAIN DE POIVRE   peppercorn
GRAINE DE MOUTARDE   mustard seed
HOUX   holly
HUILE   cooking oil
HUILE D'AMANDE   almond oil
HUILE D'ARACHIDE   peanut oil
HUILE D'OLIVE   olive oil
HUILE DE MAÏS   corn oil

HUILE DE NOIX   walnut oil
HUILE DE SOJA   soya bean oil
HUILE DE TOURNESOL   sunflower oil
KARI   curry
LAURIER   bay leaves
MARJOLAINE   marjoram, an herb
MAYONNAISE   dressing of egg yolks, vinegar or lemon
    juice
MENTHE POIVRÉE   peppermint
MUSCADE   nutmeg
NÉROLI   oil extracted from the flowers of orange trees
NOIX DE MUSCADE   nutmeg
OSEILLE   sorrel, herb
PAPRICA   paprika
PAVOT   poppy seed
POIVRE BLANC   white pepper
POIVRE DE CAYENNE   red pepper
POIVRE, GRAINS DE   peppercorns
POIVRE NOIR   black pepper
ROMARIN   rosemary
SAFRAN   saffron
SAUGE   sage
SEL   salt
SERPOLET   wild thyme
SUCRE   sugar
THYM   thyme, aromatic herb
VARENNE   herb mayonnaise
VINAIGRE   vinegar

Vegetables

AIL   garlic
ALGUES   edible seaweed
ANGLAISE, À L'   boiled or steamed vegetables
ARTICHAUT   artichoke
ARTICHAUT À LA BARIGOULE   artichoke stuffed with
    meat or mushroom and salted pork

ARTICHAUT À LA CATALANE   artichoke stuffed with sautéed onion

ARTICHAUT À LA GRECQUE   artichoke cooked with herbs and olive oil

ARTICHAUT À LA VINAIGRETTE   artichoke with oil and vinegar dressing

ARTICHAUT AU NATUREL   whole boiled artichoke

ARTICHAUT CLAMART   artichoke filled with peas

ARTICHAUT FARCIS   stuffed artichoke

ARTICHAUT FORESTIER   artichoke stuffed with sautéed mushrooms

ARTICHAUT RÉCAMIER   artichoke poached in wine, stuffed with mushrooms, goose liver in cream sauce

ARTICHAUT, COEURS D'   hearts of artichokes

ASPERGE   asparagus

ASPERGE AU GRATIN   asparagus with cheese sauce, and bread crumbs

ASPERGES À LA FONTANELLE   asparagus dipped into soft-boiled eggs and melted butter

ASPERGES AU NATUREL   boiled asparagus, hot or cold

ASPERGES D'ARGENTEUIL   best white asparagus

ASPERGES SAUCE FLAMANDE   hot asparagus served with hard boiled eggs, parsley and melted butter

ASPERGES, BRANCHE D'   whole boiled asparagus

ASSIETTE DE CRUDITÉS   plate of raw vegetables with oil and vinegar

ATTEREAUX   deep fried vegetables or meat with sauce

AUBERGINE   eggplant

AUBERGINE AUX TOMATES   eggplant with tomato

AUBERGINE FARCIE ARMÉNIENNE   baked eggplant stuffed with lamb

BAGRATION   macaroni and artichoke hearts, with tomato, mayonnaise and eggs

BARBOUILLADE   artichokes and broad beans

BARBOUILLÉ   stew of eggplant, onions, peppers and tomatoes

BARDATTE   cabbage stuffed with rabbit

BELLE-HÉLÈNE   with asparagus, mushrooms and truffles
BETTERAVE   beetroot
BETTERAVE À LA CRÈME   boiled beets in cream sauce
BIARROTTE   with cepe mushrooms and potato cakes
BLETTE OR BETTE   Swiss chard
BOLET   wild mushroom, also called cepe
BOUMAINE   stewed tomatoes and eggplant with anchovies
BRANCHE   vegetables served whole
BROCOLI   broccoli
BRUNOISE, EN   tiny diced vegetables
CAPOUN   cabbage filled with rice and sausage
CAPOUN FASSUM   stuffed cabbage and sausage
CÂPRES   capers
CARDON   celery-like vegetable
CAROTTES   carrots
CAROTTES À LA FLAMANDE   creamed carrots
CAROTTES BRAISÉES AU BEURRE   carrot slivers
    braised in butter
CAROTTES CHANTILLY   creamed carrots with peas
CAROTTES ÉTUVÉES AU BEURRE   carrots braised in butter
CAROTTES GLACÉES   glazed carrots
CAROTTES VICHY   carrots glazed in butter and sugar
CASTIGLIONE   sautéed mushrooms, marrow and eggplant
CAVIAR AUBERGINE   cold eggplant puree with fish eggs
CÉLERI   celery
CÉLERI AMANDINE   celery in almond sauce
CÉLERI, BRANCHE DE   branch of celery
CÉLERI, COEURS DE   hearts of celery
CÉLERI MILANAISE   celery boiled with butter and
    grated Parmesan cheese
CÉLERI-RAVE   celery root
CÈPE   large meaty wild boletus mushroom
CÈPES À LA BORDELAISE   mushrooms sautéed in oil
CÈPES PROVENÇALE   mushrooms made with garlic and
    tomatoes
CHAMPIGNONS   mushrooms
CHAMPIGNONS À BLANC   stewed mushrooms

CHAMPIGNONS À LA GRECQUE cold mushrooms
cooked in lemon juice and olive oil
CHAMPIGNONS, CRÈME AUX mushrooms with cream
CHAMPIGNONS DE PARIS cultivated mushrooms
CHAMPIGNONS DES BOIS wild mushrooms
CHAMPIGNONS FARCIS mushrooms stuffed with
butter, cream, Swiss cheese
CHAMPIGNONS FARCIS D'ÉPINARDS mushrooms
with spinach and ham stuffing
CHAMPIGNONS FARCIS DE CRABE mushrooms with
crab meat stuffing
CHAMPIGNONS FARCIS DE DUXELLES mushrooms
with minced mushroom stuffing
CHAMPIGNONS SAUTÉS AU BEURRE mushrooms
sautéed in butter
CHAMPIGNONS SAUVAGES wild mushrooms
CHAMPIGNONS SOUS CLOCHE baked mushrooms
CHANTERELLE pale, curly wild mushroom
CHÂTAIGNE D'EAU water chestnut
CHAYOT squash
CHICORÉE curly endive
CHICORÉE AMÈRE bitter chicory
CHICORÉE FRISÉE curly leafed chicory
CHICORÉE SAUVAGE wild chicory
CHINONAISE potatoes and sausage in cabbage
CHOU cabbage
CHOU À L'AUTRICHIENNE brussels sprouts cooked
with sour cream
CHOU BLANC white cabbage
CHOU DE BRUXELLES brussels sprouts
CHOU DE CHINE Chinese cabbage
CHOU DE SAVOIE savoy cabbage
CHOU FRISÉ kale
CHOU MARIN sea kale
CHOU NAVET rutabaga
CHOU RAVE kohlrabi
CHOU ROUGE red cabbage

CHOU ROUGE À LA FLAMANDE red cabbage with apples and vinegar

CHOU ROUGE À LA LIMOUSINE stewed red cabbage with chestnuts and pork fat

CHOU ROUGE AUX MARRONS red cabbage with chestnuts

CHOU VERT curly green Savoy cabbage

CHOU VERT EN GRATIN cabbage with cheese

CHOU-FLEUR cauliflower

CHOU-FLEUR AU BEURRE NOIR cauliflower with black butter

CHOU-FLEUR PANÉ cauliflower fried in breadcrumbs

CHOU-FLEUR RISSOLÉ cauliflower boiled and sautéed in butter

CHOU-LARD cabbage cooked with bacon

CHOUCROUTE sauerkraut

CHOUCROUTE BRAISÉE ALSACIENNE braised sauerkraut

CHOUCROUTE GARNIE sauerkraut braised with meats

CHOUÉE boiled cabbage

CHOUX DE BRUXELLES brussels sprouts

CIBOULE spring onion

CIBOULETTES chives

CITROUILLE pumpkin

COEURS D'ARTICHAUTS hearts of artichokes

COEURS DE PALMIER tender hearts of palm

CONCOMBRE cucumber

CONCOMBRES PERSILLÉS À LA CRÈME parsleyed or creamed cucumbers

CORNE D'ABONDANCE brown mushroom

COULEMELLE mushroom

COULIS puree of raw or cooked vegetables or fruit

COURGE squash

COURGETTE zucchini or squash

COURGETTE NIÇOISE squash prepared with onions and tomatoes

COUSINAT stew made of ham, artichokes, carrots and green beans

CRESSON   watercress

CROUSTADE MAZAGRAN   a baked shell of mashed potatoes

CROÛTE AUX CHAMPIGNONS   creamed mushrooms in pastry shell

D'ARTAGNAN   stuffed tomato and potato croquettes

DIABLE, ARTICHAUTS À LA   sautéed spicy, stuffed artichokes

DORIA   cucumber

DUBARRY   cauliflower with cheese sauce

DUXELLES   mushrooms and shallots sautéed in butter and cream

ÉCHALOTES   shallots, like small onion with garlic flavor

ÉGYPTIENNE, À L'   served with lentils

ENDIVE BELGE   salad vegetable with crispy and bitter leaves

ENDIVE BRAISÉE   endive braised in butter with diced ham

ENDIVE BRUXELLOISE   steamed endive rolled in ham

ENDIVES   chicory

ENDIVES À LA NORMANDE   braised endives simmered in cream

ENDIVES AU JAMBON À LA SAUCE MORNAY   endives and ham, baked in cheese sauce

ENDIVES BRAISÉES À LA FLAMANDE   endives braised in butter

ENDIVES BRAISÉES MADÈRE   endives with Madeira and vegetables

ENDIVES MEUNIÈRE   sautéed endives with black butter sauce

ÉPI DE MAÏS   ear of sweet corn

ÉPINARD   spinach

ÉPINARDS À LA CRÈME   spinach braised in cream

ÉPINARDS AU JUS   spinach braised in stock

ÉPINARDS BLANCHIS   boiled spinach with melted butter

FARCIDURE   vegetable soup dumpling

FASÉOLE   kidney bean

FECHUN   stuffed cabbage

FENOUIL   fennel
FENOUIL GRATINÉ   fennel with cheese
FERMIÈRE   local produce
FEUILLES DE BETTERAVE   beet leaves
FÉVEROLES   kidney beans
FÈVES   broad beans or fava beans
FLAGEOLET   a small bean usually green in color
FLAMICHE   leek and cream tart
FLORENTINE   with spinach
FONDS D'ARTICHAUTS   artichoke bottoms
GIROLLE   wild mushroom, also called chanterelle
GIROLLE À LA PROVENÇALE   wild mushrooms
   sautéed with garlic and onions
GOMBO   okra
GOUSSE D'AIL   clove of garlic
GRATIN D'ÉPINARDS   spinach
GRECQUE, À LA   cold vegetables in seasoned oil and
   lemon juice
GRELOT   small white bulb onion
HARICOT   bean
HARICOT BEURRE   butter bean
HARICOT BLANC   white lima bean
HARICOT DE LIMA   lima bean
HARICOT D'ESPAGNE   runner bean
HARICOT MANGE-TOUT   butter bean
HARICOT ROUGE   red kidney bean
HARICOT VERT   green bean
HARICOTS VERTS À LA LYONNAISE   green beans
   cooked with onions
HARICOTS VERTS À LA PROVENÇALE   green beans
   with tomato
HARICOT VERT AU NATUREL   green string beans,
   blanched and buttered
IGNAME   yam, tropical root vegetable
JARDINIÈRE   garnish of fresh cooked vegetables
JULIENNE   slivered vegetables or meat
LAITUE   lettuce

LAITUE BRAISÉE   braised lettuce
LAITUE PAYSANNE   lettuce cooked with ham, onions
  and carrots
LANGUEDOCIENNE   tomatoes and wild mushrooms
LANGUEDOCIENNE, GRATIN À LA   baked eggplant
  with tomatoes, breadcrumbs and garlic
LÉGUME   vegetable
LÉGUMES À LA GRECQUE   marinated vegetables, Greek
  style
LENTILLE   lentil
LIMOUSINE, À LA   red cabbage, chestnuts and mushrooms
LOUBIA   dried kidney beans
MACÉDOINE DE FRUITS   diced mixed fruit or vegetables
MACÉDOINE DE LÉGUMES   salad of cooked vegetables
  in mayonnaise
MAÏS   corn
MANGE-TOUT   a green runner bean, a snow pea
MÉNAGÈRE   a preparation of onions, potatoes and carrots
MIREPOIX   cubes of carrots and onions or mixed vegetables
MORILLE   wild morel mushroom, dark brown and
  conical shaped
MOUSSERON   delicate wild spring mushroom
MOUSSERON À LA CRÈME   mushroom in cream sauce
NAVET   turnip
NAVET À LA CHAMPENOISE   turnip and onion casserole
NAVET GLACÉ   glazed turnip
NIVERNAISE, À LA   garnish of carrots, onions, potatoes
OEUF AUX AUBERGINES FRITES   egg with fried eggplant
OEUF LUCULLUS   poached egg on artichoke heart in
  cream sauce with foie gras
OIGNON   onion
OIGNONS BLANC GLACÉS   glazed white onions
ORONGE   wild mushroom
PAILLETÉ, OIGNON   fried onion rings
PANAIS   parsnip
PARISIENNE, À LA   varied vegetable garnish including
  potato balls fried and tossed in a meat glaze

PASSE-PIERRE edible seaweed

PAYSAN garnish of carrots, turnips, onions, celery and bacon

PERSANE, À LA fried eggplant, onion, peppers and tomato

PERSIL parsley

PERSILLADE chopped parsley and garlic

PETITS POIS peas

PETITS POIS À LA FRANÇAISE young peas and baby
onions

PETITS POIS FRAIS fresh peas braised with onions and
butter

PETITS POIS AU LARD peas with bacon

PETIT SALÉ AUX LENTILLES boiled bacon with lentils
in a casserole

PIMENT DOUX sweet red pimento

PIMENT VERT green pimento

PISSALADIÈRE Provençale onion and anchovy pie

PLEUROTE wild mushroom

POINTES D'ASPERGES asparagus tips

POIREAU leek

POIREAU À LA NIÇOISE leek stewed with oil and
tomatoes

POIS pea

POIS À LA FRANÇAISE green peas cooked with onions
and lettuce

POIS CASSÉS split peas

POIS CHICHE chick pea

POIS FRAIS, BRAISAGE DE fresh peas, braised lettuce
and scallions

POIVRON green or red pepper

POIVRON FARCIS AU RIZ pepper stuffed with rice

POLENTA cooked cornmeal, water, butter and cheese

POTIRON pumpkin

PRINTANIÈRE with vegetable garnish

PURÉE DE LÉGUME finely creamed vegetable

PURÉE SOUBISE creamed onions

PURÉE ST. GERMAIN creamed green peas

QUICHE tart with egg and cream, meat or vegetable filling

RACLETTE   melted cheese with boiled potatoes, pickles and pickled onions

RADIS   radish

RAIFORT   horseradish

RATATOUILLE   stewed squash, tomatoes, vegetables and garlic

RATATOUILLE NIÇOISE   eggplant, onions, tomatoes and peppers stewed in oil

RHUBARBE   rhubarb

SALADE RUSSE   cooked vegetables in mayonnaise

SALPICON   diced vegetables, meat and/or fish in a sauce

SCAROLE   escarole

SOISSONS, HARICOTS DE   dried or fresh white beans

SOUBISE   puree of onions and rice

SOUFFLÉ DE LÉGUMES   puree of cooked vegetables

ST-GERMAIN   with peas

TARTE À L'OIGNON   onion tart

TARTE À LA TOMATE   custard and tomato pie

TARTE AUX ÉPINARDS   pastry shell filled with creamed spinach

TERRINE   earthenware container for baking meat, game, fish or vegetable mixture

TIAN   vegetable mixture cooked in an earthenware dish

TIMBALE D'ÉPINARDS   molded spinach custard

TOMATE   tomato

TOMATE À L'ANTIBOISE   marinated tomato stuffed with tuna

TOMATE GRILLÉE   grilled tomato

TOMATE POLONAISE   breaded baked tomato

TOMATE PROVENÇALE   tomato with breadcrumbs and garlic

TOPINAMBOUR   Jerusalem artichoke

TRUFFE   truffle, in the onion family, used for flavoring

VICHY   a brand of mineral water

VRILLES DE LA VIGNE   vine cuttings, usually prepared with olive oil

ZEWELMAI   onion and cream flan

Wines, Beers, and Liquors

AMER PICON   aperitif of orange with quinine added to white wine or beer

APÉRITIF   wine and brandy with herbs and bitters, e.g., Byrrh, Dubonnet, Pastis, Pernod

APPELLATION D'ORIGINE CONTRÔLÉE (A.O.C.)   wine checked by the government to insure proper description

ARMAGNAC   brandy distilled from wine

BEAUJOLAIS   red wine, e.g., Brouilly, Chenas, Chiroubles, Côte de Brouilly, Fleurie, Juliénas, Morgon, Moulin-à-Vent, Saint-Amour

BÉNÉDICTINE   green brandy with herb and orange flavoring

BIÈRE   beer

BIÈRE BLONDE   ale, light lager

BIÈRE BRUNE   stout, dark lager beer

BIÈRE EN BOUTEILLE   bottled beer

BIÈRE PRESSION   beer on tap

BIÈRE, UN DEMI   8 ozs. beer

BOISSON   drink

BORDEAUX   wines made in the Bordeaux region, e.g., Médoc, Grave, Pomerol, Saint Emilion

BROU DE NOIX   walnut liqueur

BRUT   dry in wines, unsweetened

BRUT ZÉRO   no sugar

BYRRH   aperitif of red wine and quinine

CALVADOS   apple brandy

CARTE DES VINS   wine list

CAVE   wine cellar or wine shop

CÉPAGE   grape type

CHABLIS   white wine

CHAI   wine storeroom

CHARTREUSE   herb and spiced liqueur

CHÂTEAU   castle

CHOPE   tankard

CLAIRET   very light red wine

CLARET   red wine
CLOS   vineyard
COINTREAU   orange liqueur
CORDIAL   a sweet alcoholic drink
CORSE   Corsica
CRÉMANT   semi-sparkling
CRÈME DE CACAO   cocoa liqueur
CRÈME DE CASSIS   blackcurrant liqueur
CRU   raw, also system of grading wine; premier cru,
   grand cru, cru classé, in descending order
CURAÇAO   liqueur from orange peel
CUVÉE   blend of wine
DEMI   half, also a glass of beer
DEMI-SEC   sweet
DIGESTIF   after-dinner liqueur
DOMAINE   estate
DOSAGE   amount of sugar added to champagne,
   proportioning, measure
DUBONNET   wine-based aperitif
EAU-DE-VIE   spirits, like brandy
EXTRA-SEC   very dry
FRAMBOISE   raspberry, also raspberry liqueur
GIN-TONIQUE   gin and tonic, the mixed drink
GRAND CRU   wine of exceptional quality
GRAND MARNIER   orange liqueur
GUEUZELAMBIC   Flemish bitter beer
HOUBLON   hops
HYPOCRAS   spiced red wine
IZARRA   liqueur similar to Chartreuse
JEREZ   Spanish sherry
KIR   white wine mixed with black currant liqueur
KIR ROYAL   champagne mixed with black currant
   liqueur
KIRSCH   cherry liqueur
KUMMEL   caraway seed liqueur
MAÎTRE DE CHAI   master in charge of wine making
MARC   type of brandy

MARC DE BOURGOGNE   brandy distilled from pressed grape skins and seeds

MILLÉSIME   year of the wine

MIRABELLE   brandy from yellow plums

MIS EN BOUTEILLES AU CHÂTEAU   bottled at the château

MOELLEUX   mellow sweet wines

MOUSSEUX   sparkling or frothy

MUSCADET   white wine

MUSCAT   dessert wine

NOILLY PRAT   vermouth

PASTIS   anise flavored alcohol like Pernod and Ricard

PERLANT   slightly sparkling

PERNOD   before-dinner drink which tastes like Absinthe

PÉTILLANT   slightly sparkling

PINEAU DES CHARENTES   sweet wine

PIPPERMINT GET   bright green alcoholic mint drink

POIRE WILLIAMS   pear brandy

PORTO   port

PRESSION, BIÈRE   draft beer

QUETSCH   liquor distilled from plums

RANCIO   dessert wine

RHUM   rum

RICARD   aperitif of wine with aniseed, like Pernod

SANTÉ! (À VOTRE)   cheers

ST-RAPHAEL   quinine flavored aperitif

SUPÉRIEUR   high alcohol content

SUZE   bitter liqueur

TASTE-VIN   wine tasting cup

TIRE-BOUCHON   corkscrew

TRIPLE SEC   orange liqueur

V.S.O.P. VERY SPECIAL OLD PALE   cognac aged 5 years

VIGNOBLE   vineyard

VIN   wine

VIN BLANC   white wine

VIN CHAMBRÉ   wine at room temperature

VIN CONSOMMATION COURANTE   plain table wine

VIN DE TABLE   plain table wine
VIN DOUX   dessert wine
VIN DOUX NATUREL   sweet wine
VIN DU PAYS   local wine
VIN GRIS   pale red-pink wine
VIN LIMITE QUALITÉ SUPÉRIEURE VDQS   second
   category wine
VIN MAISON   house wine
VIN MOUSSEUX   sparkling wine
VIN ORDINAIRE   everyday table wine
VIN ROSÉ   pink wine
VIN ROUGE   red wine
VIN SEC   dry wine
XÉRÈS   sherry

4

What It Means: A Complete Alphabetical Dictionary of French Food and Drink

A

À LA   in the fashion of
À POINT   medium rare
ABAISSE   rolled pastry
ABATS   organ meats
ABATTIS   giblets of fowl
ABLETTE   bleak, a freshwater fish
ABRICOT   apricot
ACIDULÉ   acidic, as tart lemon candy
ACTINIE   sea anemone
ADDITION   your bill
AEGLE   hybrid tangerine/grapefruit (ugli fruit)
AFRICAINE   with eggplant, mushrooms, potatoes and tomatoes
AGNEAU   lamb
AGNEAU, BARON D'   saddle and hind legs of lamb
AGNEAU, CARRÉ D'   rack, rib chops or cutlets of lamb
AGNEAU, CÔTELETTE D'   cutlet or lamb chop
AGNEAU: PRÉ-SALÉ   salt-marsh lamb
AGNEAU, EPAULE D'   shoulder of lamb
AGNEAU, FILET MIGNON D'   small, boned cutlet of lamb
AGNEAU, GIGOT D'   leg of lamb
AGNEAU, LAIT   milk fed lamb
AGNEAU, MÉDAILLON D'   small, boned cutlet of lamb

AGNEAU, NOISETTE D'   small, boned, finest cut cutlet of lamb

AGNEAU PERSILLÉ   baked leg of lamb larded with pork fat, garlic, wine, parsley

AGNEAU POITRINE D'   breast of lamb

AGNEAU, SELLE D'   saddle of lamb

AGNÈS SOREL   quiche made with cream and cheese

AGRUMES   citrus fruits

AIGLEFIN   fresh haddock

AIGO BOUIDO   garlic soup over bread, sprinkled with cheese

AIGO SAU   fish soup with potatoes, garlic, tomato, parsley, onion, bay leaf

AIGRE   sour

AIGRE-DOUX   sweet and sour

AIGRELETTE   tart sauce

AIGRETTE   cheese fritter

AIGUILLETTE   a thin strip of poultry or meat

AIGUILLETTE DE CANETON   breast of duckling strips

AIL   garlic

AIL, SOUPE À   garlic and milk soup, served with cheese

AILE   wing of poultry or game bird

AILERON   wing tip

AILLADE   bread rubbed with oil and garlic

AIRELLE   cranberry

AIRELLE ROUGE   cranberry

AISY CENDRÉ   firm, fruity cheese, covered in ash

ALCOOL   alcohol

ALÉNOIS   watercress

ALGUES   edible seaweed

ALICOT   fowl wings and giblets stewed with chestnuts (Périgord)

ALIGOT   mashed potatoes with fresh Cantal cheese and garlic

ALIMENT POUR ENFANTS   baby food

ALIMENTATION   food shop

ALL CRÉMAT   sauce made with garlic and olive oil for fish (Languedoc)

ALLELUIA   little cake

ALLEMANDE   with noodles and mashed potatoes

ALLEMANDE SAUCE   cream sauce of egg yolks and lemon juice

ALLUMETTES   fried shoestring potatoes or pastry strips

ALOSE   shad

ALOSE À LA CRÊME   shad in cream sauce

ALOSE ADOUR   herring stuffed and baked with ham

ALOSE AU FOUR   baked shad

ALOSE AVIGNONNAISE   fried shad, baked with sorrel

ALOSE LOIRE   shad broiled, then baked over sorrel

ALOUETTE   lark; also a lamb dish made with shoulder, curry and cream

ALOUETTE SANS TÊTE   sliced veal rolled and stuffed with meat

ALOYAU   sirloin of beef

ALPHÉE   prawn-like shellfish

ALSACIENNE   with sauerkraut, ham and sausages

AMANDE   almond

AMANDE DE MER   a small clam

AMER PICON   aperitif of orange with quinine added to white wine or beer

AMOURETTES   bone marrow of calf or ox

AMUSE-GUEULE   appetizer

ANANAS   pineapple

ANANAS MELBA   pineapple on vanilla ice cream with raspberry sauce

ANCHOÏADE   mashed anchovies on toast

ANCHOIS   anchovy

ANCIENNE, À L'   cream sauce with mushrooms and wine

ANDALOUSE   with green peppers, eggplant and tomatoes

ANDOUILLE   chitterling sausage

ANDOUILLE DE VIRE   smoked pork and tripe sausage

ANDOUILLETTE   small chitterling sausage

ANETH   dill

ANETH DOUX   fennel

ANGES CHEVAL   grilled oysters with bacon

ANGLAISE, À L'   boiled or steamed vegetables

ANGUILLE   eel

ANGUILLE AU VERT   eel braised in green sauce

ANGUILLE FUMÉE   smoked eel

ANIS   anise

ANTIBOISE, À L'   with cheese, garlic, tomatoes and sardines or anchovy or tuna

ANTILLAISE   cooked in rum

APÉRITIF   wine and brandy with herbs and bitters, e.g., Byrrh, Dubonnet, Pastis, Pernod

APPELLATION D'ORIGINE CONTRÔLÉE (A.O.C.)   wine checked by the government to insure proper description

ARACHIDE   peanut

ARAIGNÉE DE MER   spider crab

ARCACHON, HUÎTRE D'   oyster with a strong flavor

ARCHIDUC   with cream and paprika

ARGENTEUIL, CRÈME   asparagus soup

ARIÉGEOISE   with cabbage, pork, potatoes, beans

ARLÉSIENNE   with eggplant, olives, onions, potatoes, rice and tomatoes

ARMAGNAC   brandy distilled from wine

ARMENONVILLE   sauce of potatoes, tomatoes and artichokes

AROMATES   spices and herbs

ARRÊTEZ   stop

ARTÉSIENNE   cooked in beer

ARTICHAUT   artichoke

ARTICHAUT À LA BARIGOULE   artichoke stuffed with meat or mushroom and salted pork

ARTICHAUT À LA CATALANE   stuffed with sautéed onion

ARTICHAUT À LA GRECQUE   artichokes cooked with herbs and olive oil

ARTICHAUT À LA VINAIGRETTE   artichoke with oil and vinegar dressing

ARTICHAUT AU NATUREL   whole boiled artichoke

ARTICHAUT CLAMART   filled with peas

ARTICHAUT FARCI   stuffed artichoke

ARTICHAUT FORESTIER   stuffed with sautéed mushrooms

ARTICHAUT RÉCAMIER   artichoke poached in wine, stuffed with mushrooms, goose liver in cream sauce

ARTICHAUT, COEURS D'   hearts of artichokes

ARTOIS   cooked in beer

ASCENSEUR   lift

ASIMINU   fish soup

ASPERGE   asparagus

ASPERGE AU GRATIN   with cheese sauce, and bread crumbs

ASPERGES À LA FONTANELLE   dipped into soft-boiled eggs and melted butter

ASPERGES AU NATUREL   boiled asparagus, hot or cold

ASPERGES D'ARGENTEUIL   best white asparagus

ASPERGES SAUCE FLAMANDE   hot asparagus served with hard boiled eggs, parsley and melted butter

ASPERGES, BRANCHE D'   whole boiled asparagus

ASPIC   any jellied dish

ASPIC DE VEAU   veal in aspic

ASSIETTE   plate

ASSIETTE ANGLAISE   platter of assorted cold cuts or cold meats

ASSIETTE CHARCUTERIE   plate of dried sausage and pâté

ASSIETTE CREUSE   soup plate

ASSIETTE DE CRUDITÉS   plate of raw vegetables with oil and vinegar

ASSIETTE DE FRUITS DE MER   seafood platter

ASSIETTE DE PÊCHEUR   assorted fish platter

ASSIETTE DE VIANDES FROIDES   cold cuts of meat

ASSIETTE SALAMI   plate of various salamis

ASSORTI   assorted

ATHERINE   fried smelt

ATTENDRI   tenderized

ATTEREAUX   deep fried vegetables or meat with sauce

AUBERGE   country inn

AUBERGINE   eggplant

AUBERGINE AUX TOMATES   eggplant with tomato

AUBERGINE FARCIE ARMÉNIENNE   baked eggplant
    stuffed with lamb

AUMONIÈRE   filled thin crepe

AURORE   tomato and cream sauce

AURORE, OEUF À L'   stuffed egg, grated cheese, with
    tomato sauce

AUTRICHIENNE   with cabbage, caraway seeds and
    paprika

AVELINE   filbert nut, hazelnut

AVOCAT   avocado

AVOCETTE   pigeon size bird similar to a wild duck

AVOINE   oats

AVOINE, FARINE D'   oatmeal

AZYME   unleavened bread

AÏOLI   garlicky blend of eggs and olive oil

B

BABA AU RHUM   spongecake with rum syrup

BABEURRE   buttermilk

BADÈCHE   sea bass

BAECKENOFE   beef, mutton, pork stewed in wine and
    potatoes

BAGRATION   macaroni and artichoke hearts, with
    tomato, mayonnaise and eggs

BAGRATION, SOUPE   veal or fish soup with macaroni

BAGUETTE   crusty white bread loaf

BAGUETTE ANCIENNE   sourdough loaf

BAGUETTE AU LEVAIN   sourdough loaf

BAIES   berries

BAIES ROSES   pink peppercorns
BALLOTTINE   poultry, boned, stuffed and rolled
BALVET   soup of pureed peas
BANANE   banana
BANANES SPLIT AU CHOCOLAT   banana with ice cream and chocolate sauce
BANON   soft mild cheese, nutty taste, from goat or sheep milk
BAR   bass
BAR DE MER   sea bass
BAR POCHÉ AU BEURRE BLANC   poached bass with white butter sauce
BAR RAYÉ   striped bass
BAR-LE-DUC   currant jelly
BARAQUILLE   triangular pastry filled with game
BARBE-DE-CAPUCIN   wild endive
BARBEAU   variety of carp
BARBEREY   mild, skimmed milk cheese
BARBOTÉ   duck
BARBOTINE   aromatic herb
BARBOUILLADE   artichokes and broad beans
BARBOUILLE   stew of eggplant, onions, peppers and tomatoes
BARBUE   brill, a Mediterranean flatfish related to turbot
BARDATTE   cabbage stuffed with rabbit
BARON   hindquarters and legs of lamb
BARQUETTE   pastry shell with various fillings
BARQUETTE ÉCOSSAISE   pastry shell with smoked salmon
BARQUETTE OSTENDAISE   pastry shells with creamed oysters
BASILIC   basil
BASQUAISE   with ham and tomatoes or red peppers
BATAVIA   type of lettuce
BATELIÈRE   pastry shells with seafood filling
BAUDROIE   monkfish
BAVAROIS   cream dessert with flavorings and custard

BAVAROIS À L'ORANGE   orange flavored Bavarian
cream dessert

BAVETTE   skirt steak

BÉARNAISE   sauce of egg yolks, butter, shallots, tarragon,
white wine, vinegar and herbs

BEAUHARNAIS   tournedos in béarnaise sauce with
artichoke hearts, potato balls and mushrooms

BEAUJOLAIS   red wine, e.g. Brouilly, Chenas, Chiroubles,
Côte de Brouilly, Fleurie, Juliénas, Morgon, Moulin-à-
Vent, Saint-Amour

BEAUMONT   buttery version of Camembert

BÉCASSE   woodcock

BÉCASSINE   snipe

BECFIGUE   bird usually grilled on a skewer

BÉCHAMEL   white sauce with butter, flour, milk and
onion

BEIGNET   fritter or doughnut

BEIGNET DE POISSON   miniature fish balls

BEIGNET ESCURES   pear fritters fried with cream

BEIGNET NIÇOIS   batter fried pieces of tunafish

BEIGNET SOUFFLÉ   fritter with fish or meat filling

BEIGNET VIENNOIS   deep-fried pastry filled with cream,
custard or jam

BELLE COMTOISE   veal with crumbs, baked with cheese
and ham

BELLE-ANGEVINE   pear

BELLE-DIJONNAISE   with black currants

BELLE-GARDE   peach

BELLE-HÉLÈNE   with asparagus, mushrooms and truffles

BELLE-HÉLÈNE, POIRE   poached pear with ice cream
and hot chocolate sauce

BELLETOILE TRIPLE-CRÈME   rich, young cheese

BELON   oysters

BELONS, DEMI-DOUZAINE DE   a half dozen oysters

BELONS, DOUZAINE DE   a dozen oysters

BELUGA   caviar

BÉNÉDICTINE   green brandy with herb and orange flavoring

BERAWECKA   fruit cake

BERCY   meat stock with flour, butter and white wine

BERGAMOTE   fruit related to oranges

BERLINGOT   candy with nuts and fruits inside

BERRICHONNE   cooked or served in blood sauce

BESI   beef jerky

BETTERAVE   beetroot

BETTERAVE À LA CRÈME   boiled beets in cream sauce

BEUGNON   sweet fritter

BEURRE   butter

BEURRE À L'ORANGE   orange butter for crepes

BEURRE AU CITRON   lemon butter

BEURRE BLANC   sauce of vinegar, shallots and butter

BEURRE CHIVRY   herb butter

BEURRE CLARIFIÉ   clarified butter

BEURRE DE CREVETTES   shrimp butter

BEURRE GASCOGNE   garlic butter

BEURRE MAÎTRE D'HÔTEL   lemon butter with chopped parsley

BEURRE MANIÉ   paste of flour and butter

BEURRE NOIR   sauce of browned butter, lemon juice or vinegar

BEURRE NOISETTE   lightly browned butter

BEURRE POUR ESCARGOTS   butter, shallot, garlic, and seasoning

BEURRE RAIFORT   horseradish butter

BEURRE VIERGE   butter sauce with salt, pepper and lemon juice

BEURSAUDES   bacon or pork fried, then baked

BIARROTTE   with cepe mushrooms and potato cakes

BICHE   female deer

BIÈRE   beer

BIÈRE BLONDE   ale, light lager

BIÈRE BRUNE   stout, dark lager beer

BIÈRE EN BOUTEILLE bottled beer

BIÈRE PRESSION beer on tap

BIÈRE, UN DEMI 8 ozs. beer

BIFTECK beefsteak

BIFTECK À L'ALLEMANDE hamburger

BIFTECK À L'HAMBOURGEOISE hamburger

BIFTECK AU POIVRE pepper steaks

BIFTECK MARCHAND DE VIN steak sautéed with red wine

BIGARADE orange sauce

BIGARREAU red, firm-fleshed variety of cherry

BIGNON sweet fritter

BIGORNEAU winkle, a small sea mollusk

BIJANE cold wine and bread soup

BISCOTTE rusk biscuit

BISCUIT biscuit

BISCUIT AU BEURRE butter spongecake

BISCUIT CUILLÈRE ladyfingers

BISCUIT DE REIMS small macaroon

BISCUIT DE SAVOIE spongecake

BISCUIT GLACÉ cracker or biscuit with icing on top

BISCUIT ROULÉ À L'ORANGE ET AUX AMANDES
  orange and almond sponge sheet cake

BISQUE shellfish soup

BISQUE D'ÉCREVISSES crayfish soup

BISQUE DE CREVETTES shrimp bisque

BISQUE DE HOMARD lobster chowder

BISTORTO brioche baked in ring containing aniseed

BISTRO small, atmospheric, family-run type of cafe

BITOK ground beef and onions in croquette shape

BITOKE French hamburger

BLANC DE VOLAILLE boned breast of fowl

BLANCHAILLE whitebait fish, like a sprat

BLANCHAILLE FRITE fried whitebait fish

BLANCHI blanched

BLANQUETTE veal, lamb, chicken, seafood in white sauce

BLANQUETTE D'AGNEAU   lamb stew with mushrooms and onions

BLANQUETTE DE VEAU   veal stew with onions and mushrooms

BLANQUETTE DE VEAU À L'ANCIENNE   veal cutlets sautéed with onions, carrots, mushrooms, heavy cream

BLÉ   wheat

BLETTE OR BETTE   Swiss chard

BLEU DE BRESSE   strong, salty, fermented, tangy cheese

BLEU DE SAINTE-FOY   crumbly, blue-veined cheese with a sharp taste

BLEU DE SASSENAGE   soft, blue-veined cheese with sharp taste

BLEU, AU   blood rare, usually for steak

BLINI   thick pancake eaten with caviar

BLINIS AU CAVIAR   thin buckwheat pancakes filled with caviar

BOEUF   beef

BOEUF À L'ARLÉSIENNE   beef stewed with tomatoes, eggplant, onions and olive oil

BOEUF BOUILLI   boiled beef

BOEUF BOURGUIGNON   beef stewed with red wine, onions and mushrooms

BOEUF BRAISÉ   braised beef

BOEUF EN DAUBE   marinated beef stewed in wine and vegetables

BOEUF GROS SEL   boiled beef with vegetables and coarse salt

BOEUF MIROTON   sautéed and baked beef with tomato sauce and sour pickles

BOEUF MODE EN GELÉE   jellied braised beef

BOEUF SALÉ   corned beef or salt beef

BOEUF, BAVETTE DE   skirt or flank steak

BOHÉMIENNE   with fried potatoes, olives, mushrooms

BOISSON   drink

BOISSON COMPRISE   drink included

BOISSON NON-COMPRISE   drink not included

BOITELLE   cooked with mushrooms

BOLET   wild mushroom, also called cepe

BOLOGNAISE   sauce of tomatoes and vegetables, heavy
garlic

BOMBE   molded frozen dessert

BOMBE AÏDA   tangerine ice with vanilla and kirsch

BOMBE ALHAMBRA   strawberry and vanilla layered ice
cream

BOMBE DAME-BLANCHE   vanilla ice cream with
almond mousse

BOMBE FAVORITE   meringue, apricot cream and rum,
frozen and served with chestnut puree

BOMBE MÉDICIS   ice cream with pear ice, peach mousse
and kirsch

BOMBE VÉRONIQUE   pistachio and chocolate ice cream
with grapes

BON APPÉTIT   Have a good meal; enjoy your meal

BON-CHRÉTIEN   cooked pear

BONBON   sweet or candy

BONITE   bonita, similar to tunafish

BONNE FEMME   garnish of bacon, potatoes, mushrooms
and onions

BONNE FEMME, CUISINE   home style cooking

BONNE FEMME, POTAGE   potato, carrot and leek soup

BONVALET   almond cake with ice cream

BORDEAUX   wines made in the Bordeaux region, e.g.,
Médoc, Grave, Pomerol, Saint Emilion

BORDELAISE   brown sauce of shallots, red wine and
bone marrow

BORSCHT   beet soup, Russian style

BOUC   male goat

BOUCHÉE   individual puff pastry shells

BOUCHÉE À LA FINANCIÈRE   chicken and lambs'
brains in creamy, sherry sauce

BOUCHÉE À LA REINE   pastry shells with mushrooms,
tongue and chicken

BOUCHÉE AU FROMAGE   pastry shell with cheese

BOUCHÉE DUCHESSE   mashed potatoes with mushrooms and creamed chicken, baked

BOUDIN   sausage

BOUDIN BLANC   white sausage of veal, chicken or pork

BOUDIN BLANC QUERCYNOIS   white pudding made with chicken and veal

BOUDIN DE VEAU   veal and bacon sausage

BOUDIN NOIR   pork blood sausage

BOUDIN POMMES REINETTE   blood pudding with apples

BOUFFI   smoked kipper

BOUILLABAISSE   fish stew soup

BOUILLABAISSE ÉPINARDS   spinach soup with potatoes, served on bread with poached eggs

BOUILLABAISSE MARSEILLAISE   Mediterranean fish chowder with onions, leeks, olive oil, tomatoes, garlic

BOUILLI   boiled

BOUILLITURE D'ANGUILLES   eels stewed in wine

BOUILLON   a light soup or broth (also see consommé)

BOULE   ball, or round loaf

BOULE-DE-NEIGE   ice cream covered with whipped cream

BOULES DE NEIGE AU CHOCOLAT   snowballs of egg whites and chocolate

BOULETTE   meatball or fishball

BOULETTE D'AVESNES   cheese with strong taste and smell, from cow's milk

BOUMAINE   stewed tomatoes and eggplant with anchovies

BOUQUET   large reddish shrimp

BOUQUET GARNI   bag of herbs cooked in stew or soup

BOURDALOUE   fruit cooked in a light syrup

BOURDANE   apple dumpling

BOURDELOT   apple baked in pastry

BOURDELOT POIRES   baked pears

BOURGEOISE, À LA   braised meat, family style

BOURGUIGNON, POTAGE   heavy vegetable soup with sausage and pork

BOURGUIGNONNE, À LA   with red wine, onions, mushrooms and bacon

BOURIBOT   spicy duck stew with red wine

BOURRIDE   garlicky fish stew

BOURRIDE À L'AÏOLI   fish stew with garlic mayonnaise, from Provence

BOURSAULT   rich, mild, nutty flavor soft cheese

BOURSIN TRIPLE-CRÈME   dessert cheese

BRAISER   braise in a covered pan at low temperature

BRANCHE   vegetables served whole

BRANDADE DE MORUE   creamed salt cod

BRAOU BOUFFAT   soup of rice and cabbage

BRASSERIE   cafe restaurant open late hours

BREBIS   sheep

BRÈME   bream; a carp fish

BRESI   dried, smoked beef in thin slices

BRESSAN   goat's cheese with a slight goaty smell

BRESSE, BLEU DE   blue-veined cheese from cow's milk

BRETON, GÂTEAU   rich cake

BRETONNE   sauce of wine, carrots, leeks and celery

BRETZEL   pretzel

BRIE   soft paste cheese with delicate flavor

BRIE DE MEAUX   soft, mild, fermented cheese

BRIGNE   sweet fritter

BRIGNOLE   dried plum

BRIOCHE   sweet roll

BRISOLETTE   a very small cocktail appetizer or hors d'oeuvre

BROCCANA   sausage-meat and veal pâté

BROCHE, EN   roasted on a skewer, usually over an open fire

BROCHET   pike

BROCHET BADOISE   baked pike cooked with sour cream

BROCHETTE   meat or fish and vegetables on a skewer

BROCHETTE JURASSIENNE   pieces of cheese wrapped in ham and fried

BROCOLI   broccoli

BROU   soup made from cabbage and rice

BROU DE NOIX   walnut liqueur

BROUFADE   beef and onion stew with anchovies and capers

BROUILLÉ   scrambled

BROUSSE VÉSUBIE   soft and very mild cheese

BROYÉ   cereal cake used for dessert

BRUGNON   nectarine

BRÛLÉ   burned or caramelized

BRUN   browned before poaching or braising

BRUNOISE, EN   tiny diced vegetables

BRUT   dry in wines, unsweetened

BRUT ZÉRO   no sugar

BRUXELLOIS, POTAGE   Brussels sprout soup

BUERRE DE CACAHOUÈTES   peanut butter

BUFFET   station restaurant or bar/restaurant in a hotel

BUFFET FROID   dishes served cold from a buffet

BUGNE   sweet fritter

BULOT   large sea snail

BYRRH   aperitif of red wine and quinine

C

CABÉCOU   small round goat cheese

CABILLAUD   codfish

CABILLAUD AU FOUR   baked codfish

CABILLAUD BONNE FEMME   wine poached codfish in creamy sauce

CABRI   kid goat

CACAHOUÈTES   peanuts

CACAO   cocoa

CACCAVELLI   lemon cheesecake

CACHER   kosher

CACHUSE   braised pork

CAFÉ   coffee
CAFÉ ALLONGÉ   weak espresso
CAFÉ AU LAIT   espresso with warmed or lightly steamed milk
CAFÉ COMPLET   continental breakfast; coffee with hot milk, rolls, butter, jam
CAFÉ CRÈME   espresso with warmed or lightly steamed milk
CAFÉ DÉCAFÉINÉ   decaffeinated coffee
CAFÉ EN POUDRE   instant powder coffee
CAFÉ EXPRESS   plain black espresso
CAFÉ FILTRE   filtered American style coffee
CAFÉ FRAPPÉ   iced coffee
CAFÉ GLACÉ   coffee flavored ice cream dessert
CAFÉ GRAND   large cup of coffee
CAFÉ LIÉGEOIS   iced coffee with ice cream and whipped cream
CAFÉ NATURE   black coffee
CAFÉ NOIR   small black coffee
CAFÉ SANS CAFÉINE   caffeine free coffee
CAFÉ SERRÉ   extra strong espresso
CAFÉ SOLUBLE   instant coffee
CAGOUILLES VIGNERONNE   snails cooked in white wine
CAÏEU   giant mussel
CAILLE   quail
CAILLÉ   clotted or curdled
CAILLETTE   pork liver and bacon croquette
CAION   pork
CAISSE   cash register
CAJASSE   sweet, rum cake
CAJASSE SARLADAISE   rum flavored pastry
CAJOU, NOIX DE   cashew nut
CALAMAR   squid
CALISSON   marzipan sweet
CALMAR   squid
CALVADOS   apple brandy

CAMEMBERT   soft paste cheese
CAMOMILLE   camomile tea
CAMPAGNE   country
CANAPÉS   toasted bread with a variety of garnishes
CANAPÉS À LA CRÈME DE FROMAGE   cream cheese
   on toast
CANAPÉS CREVETTES   shrimp canapes
CANARD   duck
CANARD À L'ORANGE   roast duck braised with oranges
   and orange liqueur
CANARD AUX CERISES   duck with cherries
CANARD AUX OLIVES   duck cooked with olives
CANARD MONTMORENCY   duck in wine flavored jelly
   with cherries
CANARD NANTAIS   delicate flavored small duck
CANARD ROUEN   cross between domestic and wild
   duck
CANARD ROUENNAIS   duck with sauce from the blood
CANARD SAUVAGE   wild duck
CANARD VERTS POIS   steamed duckling with peas
CANCALAIS   fish consommé
CANCALAISE   oysters and shrimps in cream wine sauce
CANCOILLOTTE   skimmed milk cheese eaten warm on
   toast
CANETON   duckling
CANETON À L'ORANGE   duckling with orange
CANETON À LA BIGARADE   duckling with bitter
   oranges
CANETON AUX CERISES   duckling with cherries
CANETON AUX NAVETS   duck with turnips
CANETON AUX OLIVES   duck with olives
CANETON MONTMORENCY   roast duck with poached
   cherries in a port sauce
CANISTRELLI   almond and hazelnut cake
CANNEBERGE   cranberry
CANNELLE   cinnamon
CANNELON   puff-pastry with meat or fish filling

CANTAL   semi-hard cheese
CAPELAN   codfish
CAPILOTADE   meat hash
CAPOUN   cabbage filled with rice and sausage
CAPOUN FASSUM   stuffed cabbage and sausage
CÂPRES   capers
CÂPRES, SAUCE AUX   sauce from capers and butter
CAPRICE   a dessert
CAPRICE DES DIEUX   mild double-cream cheese
CAPUCINE   nasturtium, like caper, used in salads
CAPUCINE MUSCOVITE   appetizer of shrimp and egg
    yolks on toast
CARAFE   pitcher; house wine is often served in a carafe
CARAFE D'EAU   pitcher of tap water
CARAMEL   cooked confection
CARAMOTE   large prawn
CARBONADE   braised beef stew with beer and onions
CARBONADE DE BOEUF PROVENÇALE   casserole of
    beef, onions and potatoes
CARBONADE FLAMANDE   browned slices of beef
    cooked in beer
CARDINAL   garnish for fish, of mushrooms, truffles,
    scallops
CARDINAL, SAUCE   sauce of pieces of lobster or crayfish
CARDINALIZER   cooking shellfish in boiling salt water
CARDON   celery-like vegetable
CARGOLADE   snails
CARI   curry
CAROTTES   carrots
CAROTTES À LA FLAMANDE   creamed carrots
CAROTTES BRAISÉES AU BEURRE   carrot slivers
    braised in butter
CAROTTES CHANTILLY   creamed carrots with peas
CAROTTES ÉTUVÉES AU BEURRE   carrots braised in
    butter
CAROTTES GLACÉES   glazed carrots
CAROTTES RÂPÉES   carrot salad with vinaigrette sauce

CAROTTES VICHY   carrots glazed in butter and sugar
CARPE   carp fish
CARPE AU JUIF   boiled carp served cold in aspic
CARPE POLONAISE   carp cooked in red wine with
   onions
CARRÉ   rack
CARRÉ D'AGNEAU   rack of lamb
CARRÉ D'AGNEAU PERSILLÉ   roast lamb with parsley
CARRÉ DE PORC   rack of pork
CARRÉ DE PORC RÔTI   roast loin of pork
CARRÉ DE VEAU   rack of veal
CARRELET   flounder
CARTE   the bill of fare or menu
CARTE CONSEILLÉE   recommended or featured items
CARTE DES VINS   wine list
CARTE DU JOUR   today's bill of fare
CARVI   caraway seeds
CASSATE   ice cream dessert made with fruits
CASSE-CROÛTE   a snack
CASSE-MUSEAU   small cake
CASSEROLE   a saucepan
CASSIS   black currant
CASSISSINE   black currant sweet candy or stuffing
CASSOLETTE   a small casserole or saucepan
CASSONADE   brown sugar
CASSOULET   casserole of beans, sausages, duck, pork,
   lamb
CASSOULET DE CASTELNAUDARY   white bean stew
   with goosefat, lamb, pork
CASSOULET PÉRIGOURDIN   stew of beans, mutton and
   sausage
CASSOULET TOULOUSAIN   stew of beans, onion, pork,
   lamb, sausage, duck or goose
CASTAGNACI   chestnut pancakes
CASTAGNOLE   batter fritter
CASTIGLIONE   sautéed mushrooms, marrow and
   eggplant

CATALANE   eggplant, tomatoes, onions, peppers and rice
CATALANE, MOUTON À LA   mutton braised in wine
    with ham, vegetables and garlic
CATALANE, SAUCISSE À LA   fried sausage with garlic
CATALANE, SOUPE   tomato and onion soup
CATIGOT   eel stewed in wine and tomatoes
CAUCHOISE   white meat in cream with Calvados sauce
    and apples
CAUDIÈRE   fish stew with mussels cooked with white
    wine
CAVE   wine cellar or wine shop
CAVIAR   sturgeon eggs
CAVIAR AUBERGINE   cold eggplant puree with fish eggs
CAVIAR BLANC   mullet eggs
CAVIAR FRAIS   fresh fish eggs
CAVIAR MALOSSIL   fish eggs, lightly salted
CAVIAR NIÇOIS   anchovies, oil, fish eggs, usually served
    on toast
CAVOUR   mushrooms stuffed with chicken liver
CAYENNE   hot red pepper
CÉDRAT   sour lemon
CÉLERI   celery
CÉLERI AMANDINE   celery in almond sauce
CÉLERI, BRANCHE DE   branch of celery
CÉLERI, COEURS DE   hearts of celery
CÉLERI MILANAISE   boiled with butter and grated
    Parmesan cheese
CÉLERI-RAVE   celery root
CÉLESTINE, POTAGE   soup of leeks and potatoes
CÉLESTINE, POULARDE   sautéed chicken and mush-
    rooms in wine, cream sauce
CENDRE DES RICEYS   skimmed-milk cheese with nutty
    taste
CÉPAGE   grape type
CÈPE   large meaty wild boletus mushroom
CÈPES À LA BORDELAISE   mushrooms sautéed in oil

CÈPES, POTAGE DE   dried mushroom soup
CÈPES PROVENÇALE   mushrooms made with garlic and tomatoes
CÉREALE   cereal
CERF   venison
CERFEUIL   chervil
CERISE   cherry
CERISE NOIRE   black cherry
CERISES JUBILÉE   cherries flamed in brandy over ice cream
CERNEAU   green walnut meat
CERVELAS   sausage
CERVELAS EN BRIOCHE   pork sausage in brioche pastry
CERVELLE   brains
CERVELLE CANUT   cheese with herbs wine and vinegar
CERVELLES   brains of calf or lamb
CERVELLES AU BEURRE NOIR   sautéed brains in brown butter sauce
CÉVÉNOLE   with chestnuts and mushrooms
CHABLIS   white wine
CHABLISIENNE   cooked and served in white wine
CHABRILLAN   puree of tomato soup
CHACHLIK   lamb or beef roasted on a skewer with onions and peppers
CHADEAU   a rich dessert type sauce
CHAI   wine storeroom
CHAIR   fleshy portion of either poultry or meat
CHAIR BLANCHE   white meat
CHAMBARAND, TRAPPISTE   soft, mild and creamy cheese
CHAMOIS   wild antelope
CHAMONIX   ground chicken, hard egg in chicken broth with cream
CHAMPENOISE (POTÉE)   stew of ham, sausage and cabbage
CHAMPIGNONS   mushrooms

CHAMPIGNONS À BLANC   stewed mushrooms
CHAMPIGNONS À LA GRECQUE   cold mushrooms
cooked in lemon juice and olive oil
CHAMPIGNONS, CRÈME AUX   mushrooms with cream
CHAMPIGNONS DE PARIS   cultivated mushrooms
CHAMPIGNONS DES BOIS   wild mushrooms
CHAMPIGNONS FARCIS   mushrooms stuffed with
butter, cream, Swiss cheese
CHAMPIGNONS FARCIS D'ÉPINARDS   mushrooms
with spinach and ham stuffing
CHAMPIGNONS FARCIS DE CRABE   mushrooms with
crab meat stuffing
CHAMPIGNONS FARCIS DE DUXELLES   mushrooms
with minced mushroom stuffing
CHAMPIGNONS, POTAGE AUX   mushroom soup
CHAMPIGNONS SAUTÉS AU BEURRE   mushrooms
sautéed in butter
CHAMPIGNONS SAUVAGES   wild mushrooms
CHAMPIGNONS SOUS CLOCHE   baked mushrooms
CHAMPIGNY   pastry with apricot filling
CHANCIAU   thick pancake
CHANTERELLE   pale, curly wild mushroom
CHANTILLY   sweetened whipped cream
CHAOURCE   soft cheese with delicate, fruity taste
CHAPEAU   small round loaf of bread
CHAPELURE   breadcrumbs
CHAPON   capon or castrated chicken
CHAPON GROS SEL   capon baked in rock salt
CHARBON DE BOIS   charcoal
CHARCUTERIE   shop selling cold cuts, sausages, pâtés
CHARCUTERIE ASSORTIE   assorted pork products
CHARENTAIS   sweet melon
CHARGOUÈRE   pastry with plums or prunes
CHARIOT   cart used for hors d'oeuvres, cheese and
dessert
CHARIOT À DESSERTS   rolling cart carrying varied
desserts

CHARLOTTE   molded dessert with ladyfingers and custard filling

CHARLOTTE AUX POMMES   molded apple dessert

CHARLOTTE MALAKOFF AU CHOCOLAT   chocolate-almond cream molded in ladyfingers

CHARLOTTE RUSSE   cream custard with sponge finger cakes

CHAROLAIS   cheese from goat's milk

CHARTREUSE   herb and spiced liqueur

CHASSEUR, CONSOMMÉ   game consommé, madeira and mushrooms

CHÂTAIGNE   small chestnut

CHÂTAIGNE D'EAU   water chestnut

CHÂTEAU   castle

CHÂTEAU, ENTRECÔTE   thick sirloin steak

CHÂTEAU, POMMES   potatoes cooked in butter

CHÂTEAUBRIAND   thick fillet steak

CHAUD   hot or warm

CHAUD-FROID   poultry dish served cold with a sauce

CHAUD-FROID DE SAUMON   cold salmon in a rich jellied sauce

CHAUDE   plum tart

CHAUDEAU   orange tart

CHAUDRÉE   seafood stew

CHAUDRÉE ROCHELAISE   fish stew of tiny fish and wine

CHAUSSON   pastry shell stuffed with mussels, fish or meat

CHAUSSON AUX MOULES   turnover stuffed with mussels

CHAUSSON AUX NOISETTES   nut strudel

CHAUSSON AUX POMMES   apple turnover

CHAYOT   squash

CHEDDAR   cheese

CHEMISE, EN   wrapped with pastry

CHEVAINE OR CHEVESNE   type of carp

CHEVEUX D'ANGE   very fine pasta, like angelhair

CHÈVRE   a strong goat milk cheese
CHEVREAU   young goat
CHEVRET   goat's milk cheese with a nutty taste
CHEVREUIL   young roe deer
CHEZ NOUS, DE   speciality of the house
CHICORÉE   curly endive
CHICORÉE AMÈRE   bitter chicory
CHICORÉE FRISÉE   curly leafed chicory
CHICORÉE SAUVAGE   wild chicory
CHIFFONNADE DE CRABE   crab, eggs, mayonnaise
CHILIENNE   with rice and sweet peppers
CHINONAISE   potatoes and sausage in cabbage
CHIPIRON   small squid
CHIPOLATAS   small pork sausages
CHIVRY, SAUCE   white wine sauce with herbs
CHOCOLAT   chocolate
CHOCOLAT AMER   bittersweet chocolate
CHOCOLAT AU LAIT   milk chocolate
CHOCOLAT CHAUD   hot chocolate
CHOCOLAT EN POUDRE   cocoa
CHOIX   choice
CHOPE   tankard
CHORIZO   very spicy sausage
CHOU   cabbage
CHOU À L'AUTRICHIENNE   brussels sprouts cooked
   with sour cream
CHOU BLANC   white cabbage
CHOU DE BRUXELLES   brussels sprouts
CHOU DE CHINE   Chinese cabbage
CHOU DE SAVOIE   savoy cabbage
CHOU FARCI   stuffed cabbage
CHOU FRISÉ   kale
CHOU MARIN   sea kale
CHOU NAVET   rutabaga
CHOU RAVE   kohlrabi
CHOU ROUGE   red cabbage

CHOU ROUGE À LA FLAMANDE   red cabbage with apples and vinegar

CHOU ROUGE À LA LIMOUSINE   stewed red cabbage with chestnuts and pork fat

CHOU ROUGE AUX MARRONS   red cabbage with chestnuts

CHOU VERT   curly green Savoy cabbage

CHOU VERT EN GRATIN   cabbage with cheese

CHOU-FLEUR   cauliflower

CHOU-FLEUR AU BEURRE NOIR   cauliflower with black butter

CHOU-FLEUR PANÉ   cauliflower fried in breadcrumbs

CHOU-FLEUR RISSOLÉ   boiled and sautéed in butter

CHOU-LARD   cabbage cooked with bacon

CHOUCROUTE   sauerkraut

CHOUCROUTE BRAISÉE ALSACIENNE   braised sauerkraut

CHOUCROUTE GARNIE   sauerkraut braised with meats

CHOUÉE   boiled cabbage

CHOUX   cream puff pastry of flour, butter, water and eggs

CHOUX DE BRUXELLES   brussels sprouts

CIBOULE   spring onion

CIBOULETTES   chives

CIDRE   cider

CIGARETTE   tubular petit-four served with ice cream

CIMIER   venison hip

CINGALAISE, À LA   curried

CITEAUX   soft tangy cheese

CITRON   lemon

CITRON PRESSÉ   lemon juice with water and sugar for sweetening

CITRON VERT   lime

CITRONNADE   still lemonade

CITRONNAT   candied lemon peel

CITROUILLE   pumpkin

CITROUILLE, TARTE À LA   pumpkin pie
CIVELLES FRITES   fried baby eels
CIVET   stew of game thickened with blood
CIVET DE LANGOUSTE   lobster stewed in wine, tomatoes and onions
CIVET DE LAPIN   rabbit stewed in wine
CIVET DE LIÈVRE   hare stewed in wine
CIVET DE LIÈVRE À LA FRANÇAISE   hare cooked in wine, mushrooms and onions
CLAFOUTIS   tart of batter, fruit and black cherries
CLAFOUTIS AUX CERISES   deep-dish cherry cake
CLAIRET   very light red wine
CLAQUEBITOU   cheese with the taste of herbs and garlic
CLARET   red wine
CLÉMENTINE   tangerine
CLOCHE, SOUS   under a glass cover
CLOS   vineyard
CLOU DE GIROFLE   clove
CLOVISSE   clam
CLUPE   herring
COCA   Coca-Cola
COCHON   pig
COCHON DE LAIT   suckling pig
COCHON DE LAIT EN GELÉE   suckling pig in aspic
COCHONAILLES   sausages and pâtés served as a first course
COCO, NOIX DE   coconut
COCONS   liqueur flavored marzipan sweets
COEUR   heart
COEURS D'ARTICHAUTS   hearts of artichokes
COEURS DE PALMIER   tender palm hearts
COEUR FILET   choice cut of steak
COING   quince
COINTREAU   orange liqueur
COLBERT   dipped in egg batter, breadcrumbs and fried
COLIN   hake

COLIN À LA GRANVILLAISE   hake, like cod, served with shrimps

COLLET   mutton neck or veal

COLLIOURE, SAUCE   mayonnaise with anchovies and garlic

COLOMBE   dove

COLOMBINE   deep fried croquette with Parmesan cheese

COLONEL   lemon sherbet doused with vodka

COLVERT   wild duck

COMMANDER   to order

COMPLET   full

COMPOTE   stewed fruit

COMPOTE D'ABRICOTS   stewed fresh apricots

COMPOTE DE FRUITS   fruit poached in vanilla syrup

COMTÉ   semi-hard cheese

COMTÉ, GRUYÈRE DE   firm sharp tasting cows' milk cheese

CONCASSÉ   coarsely chopped

CONCOMBRE   cucumber

CONCOMBRE PERSILLÉ À LA CRÈME   parsleyed or creamed cucumber

CONCOMBRE, POTAGE DE   cream of cucumber soup, hot or cold

CONDÉ   rice with fruits

CONDÉ, POTAGE   mashed red bean soup

CONFISERIE   candies and confectionery

CONFIT   duck, goose, or pork preserved in its own fat

CONFIT D'OIE   goose preserved in its own fat in earthen jars

CONFIT DE CANARD   pieces of duck cooked and preserved in earthen jars

CONFITURE   jam

CONFITURE À L'ORANGE   marmalade

CONGRE   conger eel

CONSEILLÉ   recommended

CONSERVE   canned or preserved

CONSOMMATION   drinks ordered in a cafe or bar

CONSOMMÉ   clear soup

CONSOMMÉ À L'ALLEMANDE   double strength beef soup with frankfurter slices

CONSOMMÉ À L'ALSACIENNE   clear beef soup with noodles

CONSOMMÉ À L'AMÉRICAINE   double strength beef soup with green peas

CONSOMMÉ À L'IRLANDAISE   clear soup with mutton, barley and vegetables

CONSOMMÉ À L'OEUF   clear soup with a raw egg

CONSOMMÉ À LA BOUCHÈRE   clear beef soup with bone-marrow and cabbage

CONSOMMÉ À LA GAULOISE   chicken consommé with cockscombs, kidneys

CONSOMMÉ À LA PARISIENNE   chicken consommé with vegetables

CONSOMMÉ ADÈLE   clear soup with vegetables

CONSOMMÉ ALEXANDRA   clear chicken soup with chicken balls and lettuce

CONSOMMÉ AUX CHEVEUX D'ANGE   clear soup with thin noodles

CONSOMMÉ AUX VERMICELLES   clear soup with thin noodles

CONSOMMÉ BLANC   strained soup from veal and vegetables

CONSOMMÉ CANCALAIS   fish consommé with pike, oysters and parsley

CONSOMMÉ CARDINAL   clear fish soup with lobster balls

CONSOMMÉ CÉLESTINE   clear soup with chicken and noodles or crepes

CONSOMMÉ COLBERT   clear soup with poached eggs, spring vegetables

CONSOMMÉ COMMODORE   fish consommé with clams and tomatoes

CONSOMMÉ CROÛTES AU POT   beef soup, vegetables and croutons

CONSOMMÉ DE GIBIER   game soup

CONSOMMÉ DE LÉGUMES   clear soup containing vegetables

CONSOMMÉ DE POULE   chicken broth

CONSOMMÉ DE TORTUE   turtle consommé with Madeira and turtle pieces

CONSOMMÉ DE TORTUE CLAIR   turtle soup with turtle meat and sherry

CONSOMMÉ DE VOLAILLE   broth from chicken, turkey, goose, duck

CONSOMMÉ DOUBLE   double strength broth

CONSOMMÉ EN GELÉE   jellied consommé

CONSOMMÉ FLIP   consommé of leeks and ham

CONSOMMÉ JOCKEY CLUB   clear chicken soup

CONSOMMÉ JULIENNE   clear soup with shredded vegetables

CONSOMMÉ MADRILÈNE   consommé with fresh tomato and herbs

CONSOMMÉ MERCÉDÈS   chicken consommé with sherry, sliced cock's kidneys

CONSOMMÉ MONACO   chicken consommé with cheese flavored rounds

CONSOMMÉ NEMROD   game consommé with port

CONSOMMÉ ORLÉANS   chicken consommé, cream, tomato puree and pistachios

CONSOMMÉ PORTO   clear soup with port wine

CONSOMMÉ PRINCESSE   clear soup with chicken and asparagus tips

CONSOMMÉ REINE   thickened chicken consommé with strips of chicken

CONTRE-FILET   slice of steak

CONVERSATION   tart with glazing and almond filling

COPEAU DE CHOCOLAT   chocolate shavings as a cake decoration

COPPA   a variety of sausage
COQ   chicken
COQ À LA BIÈRE   chicken cooked in beer
COQ AU RIESLING   chicken in white wine and cream sauce
COQ AU VIN   chicken stewed in wine sauce
COQ DE BRUYÈRE   grouse
COQUE   small clam-like shellfish
COQUILLAGES   shellfish
COQUILLE   shell
COQUILLES-ST-JACQUES   scallops
COQUILLES-ST-JACQUES À LA MÉNAGÈRE   scallops sautéed with wine, onions, mushrooms
COQUILLES-ST-JACQUES AU GRATIN   scallops in wine with mushroom and tomato sauce
COQUILLES-ST-JACQUES BÉCHAMEL   scallops in shell with white sauce, browned
COQUILLES-ST-JACQUES CRÉOLE   scallops in wine with tomato fondue
COQUILLES-ST-JACQUES PARISIENNE   scallops and mushrooms in white wine sauce
COQUILLES-ST-JACQUES PROVENÇALE   scallops sautéed with garlic butter sauce, grated cheese, tomato, oven browned
CORBEAU   crow
CORBEILLE   basket
CORBEILLE DE FRUITS   basket of fruit
CORDE   sweet pastry
CORDIAL   a sweet alcoholic drink
CORDON BLEU, ESCALOPE   veal with ham and cheese
CORIANDRE   coriander, either fresh herbs or dried seeds
CORNE D'ABONDANCE   brown mushroom
CORNET   slice of ham or tongue rolled and stuffed; also an ice cream cone
CORNICHON   small sour pickles or gherkins
CORRÉZIENNE, GALETTE   walnut filled pastry
CORSE   Corsica

CÔTE   chop; rib
CÔTE D'AGNEAU   lamb chops
CÔTE DE BOEUF   rib steak
CÔTE DE PORC   pork chop
CÔTE DE VEAU   veal chop
CÔTE DE VEAU EN PAPILLOTE   veal chops baked in a
   parchment bag with mushrooms, onion, parsley and
   butter
CÔTELETTE   chop
CÔTELETTE D'AGNEAU   lamb cutlet
CÔTELETTE D'AGNEAU CHAMPVALLON   lamb chops
   baked in onions and potatoes
CÔTELETTES DE CHEVREUIL   venison cutlets
CÔTELETTES DE PORC AUX PRUNEAUX   pork cutlets
   with prunes
CÔTELETTES DE PORC HERBES   pork chops with herbs
CÔTELETTES NIVERNAISE   casserole of veal or pork
   chops baked with carrots, potatoes and artichoke hearts
CÔTES BLUES   large oyster
CÔTES DE BOEUF RÔTI   roast beef ribs
CÔTES DE PORC À L'AUVERGNATE   baked pork chops
   with cabbage
CÔTES DE VEAU À L'ARDENNAISE   braised veal chops
   and ham
CÔTES DE VEAU À LA BONNE FEMME   veal chops
   sautéed with onions and butter
CÔTES DE VEAU AUX HERBES   veal chops with herbs
COTRIADE   fish soup stew
COU D'OIE FARCI   stuffed goose neck
COUDENAT   pork sausage
COUKEBOOTRAM   cake with raisins
COULEMELLE   mushroom
COULIBIAC   fish in pastry baked then sliced
COULIBIAC DE SAUMON EN CROÛTE   salmon, rice
   and mushrooms baked in pastry
COULIS   puree of raw or cooked vegetables or fruit
COULOMMIERS   Brie type cheese, similar to Camembert

COUP DE JARNAC   sponge cake with jam and cognac
COUPE   dessert with ice cream and fruit
COUPE GLACÉE   sundae
COUPE JACQUES   ice cream with fruit in kirsch liqueur
COUQUE   cake
COURGE   squash
COURGETTE   zucchini or squash
COURGETTE NIÇOISE   squash prepared with onions and
    tomatoes
COURONNE   ring shaped loaf of bread
COURONNE DE RIZ AUX CREVETTES   creamed prawns
    in rice ring
COURQUIGNOISE   fish stew in white wine with mussels
COURT-BOUILLON   broth, or aromatic poaching liquid
COUSCOUS   semolina or hard wheat flour, usually
    served with a spicy lamb or chicken stew
COUSINAT   stew made of ham, artichokes, carrots and
    green beans
COUSINETTE   sour soup of sorrel, spinach, chicory and
    Swiss chard
COUTEAU   knife
COUVERT   table setting (fork, spoon, knife and plate)
COUVERT, VIN ET SERVICE COMPRIS   includes wine,
    service and table setting
COUVERT-BEURRE   cover charge including bread and
    butter
CRABE   crab
CRABE À LA PARISIENNE   crab with mayonnaise and
    chopped vegetables
CRABE À LA RUSSE   crab in the shell with mayonnaise
    and capers
CRAMIQUE   bun with currants or raisins
CRAPAUD   toad
CRAPAUDINE   poultry split and grilled
CRAPAUDINE, SAUCE   brown sauce made with onions,
    vinegar and spices

CRAQUELIN   light pastry filled with apple
CRAQUELOT   smoked, salted herring
CRÉCY   carrot soup
CRÉMANT   semi-sparkling
CRÈME   cream
CRÈME AIGRE   sour cream
CRÈME ANGLAISE   custard sauce
CRÈME ANGLAISE AU CHOCOLAT   soft chocolate custards
CRÈME ASPERGES   cream of asparagus soup
CRÈME AU BEURRE À L'ANGLAISE   custard butter cream
CRÈME AU BEURRE AU SIROP   French butter cream made with sugar syrup
CRÈME AU BUERRE À LA MERINGUE   meringue butter cream
CRÈME AUX POIREAUX   cream of leek soup
CRÈME BRÛLÉE   rich custard dessert with a top of caramelized sugar
CRÈME CARAMEL   caramel custard
CRÈME CHANTILLY   sweetened whipped cream
CRÈME D'ÉPINARDS   cream of spinach soup
CRÈME DE BOLETS   cream of boletus mushroom soup
CRÈME DE CACAO   cocoa liqueur
CRÈME DE CASSIS   black currant liqueur
CRÈME DE CÉLERI   cream of celery soup
CRÈME DE CHAMPIGNONS   cream of mushroom soup
CRÈME DE CRESSON   cream of watercress soup
CRÈME DE LAITUE   cream of lettuce soup
CRÈME DE LÉGUMES   cream of vegetable soup
CRÈME DE POULET   cream of chicken soup
CRÈME DE TOMATES   cream of tomato soup
CRÈME DE VOLAILLE   cream of chicken soup
CRÈME ÉPAISSE   thick cream
CRÈME ÉVITA   cold soup made with tomatoes and cream
CRÈME FOUETTÉ   whipped cream

CRÈME FRAÎCHE   lightly soured cream
CRÈME GLACÉE   ice cream
CRÈME HOMÈRE   egg custard with honey, wine
CRÈME MERINGUÉE   a type of egg custard decorated
    with fruits
CRÈME MOULE   baked custard dessert
CRÈME PÂTISSIÈRE   custard cream filling
CRÈME PLOMBIÈRES   custard filled with fresh fruits and
    egg whites
CRÈME RENVERSÉE   vanilla custard or flan
CRÈME SABAYON   an egg yolk and wine dessert
CRÈME VICHYSSOISE   cold potato and leek soup; very
    creamy
CRÈME VICHYSSOISE GLACÉE   iced potato and leek soup
CRÉOLE   with rice, sweet peppers and tomatoes
CRÊPE   thin pancake
CRÊPE À LA VOLAILLE   chicken pancake
CRÊPE DENTELLE   thin pancake with sweet filling
CRÊPES FARCIES JAMBON   pancakes filled with ham
    and mushrooms
CRÊPES FLORENTINES   crepes with spinach and
    mushrooms, baked with cheese sauce
CRÊPES FOURRÉES FLAMBÉES   crepes stuffed with
    orange and almonds
CRÊPES FOURRÉES GRATINÉES   filled French pancakes
CRÊPES JEANETTE   crepes filled with custard, flamed
    with brandy
CRÊPES NORMANDES   crepes with baked apple slices
    and caramel
CRÊPES POMMES DE TERRE   grated potato pancakes
CRÊPES ROULÉES FARCIES   crepes with creamed
    shellfish, gratinéed in wine and cheese sauce
CRÊPES SUZETTE   hot crepe dessert flamed with orange
    liqueur
CRÉPINETTE   small spicy flat sausage
CRÉPINETTES TRUFFÉES   pork sausages with truffles
CRESSON   watercress

CRESSON, POTAGE DE watercress soup
CRESSON, POTAGE AU watercress soup
CRÊTE DE COQ cock's comb
CRETONS fat crisps
CREUSE elongated, crinkle shelled oyster
CREVETTE shrimp
CREVETTE EN BROCHETTE shrimps broiled on skewer
CREVETTE GRISE small shrimp that turn gray when cooked
CREVETTE ROSE small shrimp that turns red when cooked
CRISTE MARINE edible algae growing on rock
CROISSANT crescent shaped roll
CROMESQUI food dipped in batter and fried
CROMESQUIS ground or chopped mixtures
CROQUANT crunchy, also small cakes made with sugar and flour
CROQUE AU SEL raw, with salt
CROQUE-MADAME toasted or fried cheese and chicken sandwich
CROQUE-MONSIEUR toasted or fried cheese and ham sandwich
CROQUEMBOUCHE crisp profiteroles filled with cream and sugar glaze
CROQUET crisp almond biscuit
CROQUETTE ground meat, fish, fowl or vegetables, coated in breadcrumbs and deep fried
CROTTIN DE CHAVIGNOL firm goat cheese
CROUSTADE pastry filled with prunes and apples
CROUSTADE DE CHAMPIGNONS pastry filled with mushrooms in a sauce
CROUSTADE DE CREVETTES NANTUA pastry with shrimp in wine sauce
CROUSTADE DE FRUITS DE MER pastry filled with seafood
CROUSTADE DE LANGOUSTES pastry shell with lobster in cream sauce

CROUSTADE DE MORILLES   morel mushrooms with
cream sauce in pastry shell
CROUSTADE DE VOLAILLE   pastry shells with a chicken
mixture
CROUSTADE JURASSIENNE   pastry shell with bacon
and cheese
CROUSTADE MAZAGRAN   a baked shell of mashed
potatoes
CROÛTE   in pastry
CROÛTE AU FROMAGE   melted cheese served over toast
CROÛTE AUX CHAMPIGNONS   creamed mushrooms in
pastry shell
CROÛTE SEL   in a salt crust
CROÛTES AU POT   cheese and bread soup
CROÛTONS   cubes of toasted or fried bread
CRU   raw, also system of grading wine; premier cru,
grand cru, cru classé, in descending order
CRUCHADE   fritter of corn meal
CRUDITÉS   raw salad vegetables
CRUSTACÉ   shellfish
CUILLER, CUILLÈRE   spoon
CUISINE BOURGEOISE   plain food
CUISINE MAIGRE   vegetarian cooking
CUISINE MINCEUR   diet cooking
CUISINE NOUVELLE   new style cooking; small portions
of light food
CUISSE   leg and thigh of poultry
CUISSE DE GRENOUILLE   frogs' legs
CUISSE DE POULET   chicken drumstick
CUISSEAU   leg of veal
CUISSON   cooking
CUISSOT   hip of venison
CUISSOT DE PORC RÔTI   roast leg of pork
CUIT   cooked
CUIT, BIEN   well-done
CULOTTE   beef rump

CULTIVATEUR, SOUPE   soup made with vegetables, pork and potatoes
CUMIN   caraway, cumin
CURAÇAO   liqueur from orange peel
CURCUMA   turmeric
CURE-DENT   toothpick
CUVÉE   blend of wine

D

D'ARTAGNAN   stuffed tomato and potato croquettes
DAGH KEBAB   veal, onions and tomatoes grilled on a skewer
DAME BLANCHE   peaches in syrup with vanilla ice cream and pineapple, in kirsch, with whipped cream
DAMES   ladies
DARBLAY   cream of potato soup
DARD   freshwater carp
DARIOLES   puff pastry shell
DARNE   slice of fish
DARNE DE SAUMON GRILLÉE   grilled salmon steak
DARNE DE SAUMON GRILLÉE AU BEURRE D'ESCARGOT   broiled salmon steak with garlic and herb butter
DARNE MONTMORENCY   salmon, mushrooms and olives
DATTE   date
DAUBE   beef stew with red wine
DAUBE DE BOEUF PROVENÇALE   casserole of beef with wine and vegetables
DAUBE MORETON   mutton stew prepared with herbs and vegetables
DAUBE PROVENÇALE   beef stew with mushrooms and onions in red wine
DAUPHIN   spicy cheese with strong smell
DAUPHINOIS, GRATIN   potatoes cooked with milk and cheese

DAURADE   sea bream

DEAUVILLAISE, SOLE À LA   poached sole with onions and cream

DÉCAFÉINÉ OR DÉCA   decaffeinated espresso

DEFARDE   stew of tripe and lambs' feet

DÉFENSE DE FUMER   no smoking

DÉJEUNER   lunch

DÉLICE   pastry for desserts

DEMI   half, also a glass of beer

DEMI SEL   soft cream cheese

DEMI-BOUTEILLE   half-bottle

DEMI-CARAPACE   half-shell

DEMI-DEUIL POULARDE   poached chicken with truffles

DEMI-GLACE   beef sauce lightened with consommé

DEMI-SEC   sweet

DEMI-TASSE   small cup of strong coffee

DEMIDOFF   chicken with pureed vegetables

DEMOISELLE   small

DEMOISELLE DE CHERBOURG   small lobster

DENT-DE-LION   dandelion

DÉPOUILLÉ   skinned or peeled

DÉSOSSÉ   boned

DIABLE   very spicy, peppery sauce

DIABLE, ARTICHAUTS À LA   sautéed spicy, stuffed artichokes

DIABLE DE MER   monkfish

DIABLE, OEUF À LA   fried egg with vinegar

DIABLE, SAUCE   sauce of vinegar, shallots and pepper

DIABLOTIN   cheese croutons served with soup

DIABOLO   lemonade

DIABOLO MENTHE   mint syrup and lemonade

DIEPPOISE, À LA   wine, mussels, shrimp, mushrooms and cream

DIGESTIF   after-dinner liqueur

DIJON   type of mustard

DIJONNAISE   made with mustard

DINDE   turkey

DINDON AUX MARRONS   turkey stuffed with chestnuts, sausage meat, pork, brandy and baked

DINDON FARCI AUX MARRONS   turkey stuffed with chestnuts

DINDON RÔTI   roast turkey

DÎNER   dinner

DIOT   pork sausage cooked in wine

DIOTS AU VIN BLANC   sausages cooked in white wine

DIPLOMATE   custard dessert with candied fruit and lady-fingers

DODINE   cold, boned stuffed duck

DODINE DE CANARD   duck stewed with onions

DODINE DE VOLAILLE   marinated chicken stuffed and braised

DOLMAS   foods wrapped in vine leaves

DOMAINE   estate

DORADE   bream

DORÉ   browned, with egg yolk

DORIA   cucumber

DOS   back

DOSAGE   amount of sugar added to champagne, proportioning, measure

DOUBLE   double

DOUBLE EXPRESS   a double cup of espresso

DOUBLE-CRÈME   cream cheese

DOUCEURS   sweets or desserts

DOUILLON   pear baked in pastry

DOUX   sweet

DRAGÉE   sugar-coated almond or sweet

DU BARRY, POTAGE   cream of cauliflower soup

DUBARRY   cauliflower with cheese sauce

DUBONNET   wine-based aperitif

DUCHESSE, POMMES DE TERRE   dish containing creamed or mashed potatoes

DUCHESSES   pastry shells with various appetizers

DUGLÈRE   tomato and herb sauce
DUXELLES   mushrooms and shallots sautéed in butter
  and cream

E

EAU   water
EAU GAZEUSE   sparkling soda water
EAU MINÉRALE   mineral water
EAU NATURELLE   water
EAU NON POTABLE   not drinking water
EAU-DE-VIE   spirits, like brandy
ÉCHALOTES   shallots, like small onion with garlic flavor
ÉCHALOTES, POTAGE AUX   onion soup made with
  shallots
ÉCHINE   spare ribs
ÉCLAIR AU CHOCOLAT   cream puff with custard cream
  filling, chocolate frosting
ÉCREVISSE   freshwater crayfish
ÉCREVISSE À LA NAGE   crayfish simmered in white
  wine, vegetables and herbs
ÉCREVISSES À LA LIÉGEOISE   crayfish with butter
  sauce
ÉGLEFIN   haddock
ÉGYPTIENNE, À L'   served with lentils
ELZEKARIA   bean and cabbage soup
ÉMINCÉ   very thin slice of meat
EMMENTAL FRANÇAIS   soft and fruity cheese
EN SUS DE   in addition
ENCORNET   small squid
ENDIVE BELGE   salad vegetable with crispy and bitter
  leaves
ENDIVE BRAISÉE   braised in butter with diced ham
ENDIVE BRUXELLOISE   steamed endive rolled in ham
ENDIVES   chicory
ENDIVES À LA NORMANDE   braised endives simmered
  in cream

ENDIVES AU JAMBON À LA SAUCE MORNAY   endives and ham, baked in cheese sauce

ENDIVES BRAISÉES À LA FLAMANDE   endives braised in butter

ENDIVES BRAISÉES MADÈRE   endives with Madeira and vegetables

ENDIVES MEUNIÈRE   sautéed endives with black butter sauce

ENTRECÔTE   beef rib steak

ENTRECÔTE CHASSEUR   steak with tomato sauce, shallots and wine

ENTRECÔTE CHÂTEAU   large thick steak

ENTRECÔTE MAÎTRE D'HÔTEL   beef rib steak with herb butter

ENTRECÔTE MARCHAND DE VIN   beef steak with wine sauce

ENTRECÔTE MINUTE   thin steak

ENTRÉE   course served after the first course but before the meat

ENTRÉE GRATUITE   entrance fee

ENTRÉE INTERDITE   no entrance

ENTREMETS   sweets

ENTREMETS CHAUDS   hot sweet dishes

ENTREMETS FROIDS   cold sweet dishes

ÉPAULE   shoulder

ÉPAULE D'AGNEAU FARCIE   stuffed shoulder of lamb

ÉPAULE DE VEAU   shoulder of veal

ÉPERLAN   smelt, fish like a large sardine

ÉPI DE MAÏS   ear of sweet corn

ÉPICE   spice

ÉPIGRAMMES D'AGNEAU ST. GERMAIN   breast of lamb wih peas

ÉPINARDS   spinach

ÉPINARDS À LA CRÈME   spinach braised in cream

ÉPINARDS AU JUS   spinach braised in stock

ÉPINARDS BLANCHIS   boiled spinach with melted butter

ÉPOISSES   soft cheese with an acid taste

ÉSAÜ   thick lentil soup

ESCALOPES   thin slices of meat

ESCALOPES À LA VIENNOISE   breaded veal cutlet

ESCALOPES DE VEAU   slices of veal

ESCALOPES DE VEAU À LA CRÈME   sliced veal with cream sauce

ESCALOPES DE VEAU BELLE COMTOISE   baked veal with cheese and ham

ESCALOPES DE VEAU GRATINÉES   casserole of veal with ham and cheese

ESCALOPES DE VEAU HOLSTEIN   veal cutlet topped with fried egg

ESCALOPES DE VEAU SAUTÉES À L'ESTRAGON   sautéed veal with tarragon

ESCARGOTS   snails

ESCARGOTS À LA BOURGUIGNONNE   snails grilled in garlic butter

ESCARGOTS À LA LANGUEDOCIENNE   snails in a spicy sauce

ESCARGOTS À LA NARBONNAISE   snails in mayonnaise and ground almonds

ESCARGOTS PETITS-GRIS   small land snails

ESCAROLE   green lettuce with slightly bitter taste

ESPADON   swordfish

ESPAGNOLE, SAUCE   vegetable, meat and tomato sauce

ESQUINADO   spider crab

ESTOFINADO   fish stew with dried cod cooked in walnut oil with eggs, garlic and cream

ESTOMAC   sheep stomach

ESTOUFFADE   stew of beef, pork, onions, mushrooms and wine

ESTOUFFADE DE BOEUF   beef with onions, wine, bacon

ESTOUFFAT   meat stewed with wine, vegetables and pork

ESTOUFFAT DE HARICOTS   stew of sausages or ham, white beans and pork

ESTRAGON   tarragon

ESTURGEON   sturgeon
ÉTOILE   star
ÉTRILLE   small crab
ÉTUVÉ   steamed
EXPLORATEUR   mild cream cheese
EXPRESS   espresso coffee
EXTRA   exceptional
EXTRA-SEC   very dry
EXTRAIT   extract

F

FAÇON   fashion or style of
FAGOT   meatball
FAGOUE   sweetbreads
FAINE   beechnut
FAISAN   pheasant
FAISAN À LA CRÈME   pheasant in cream sauce
FAISAN NORMAND   casserole of pheasant with salt
   pork, butter, apples, sour cream, pepper, applejack
FAISAN VALLÉE D'AUGE   pheasant with apples and
   cream
FAISANDÉ   aged game
FALCULELLI   cheesecake
FAMILLE   family style
FANCHETTE   cake with cream filling and meringue
FANTAISIE BOURBONNAISE   baked apricot dessert
FAR   porridge
FAR BRETON   sweet pudding with prunes
FARCE   ingredients used as stuffing
FARCE ÉVOCATION LABUFERA   rice, mushroom and
   chicken liver stuffing
FARCE FRAISES CIO-CIO-SAN   strawberry filling with
   almonds and kumquats
FARCI   stuffed
FARCIDURE   vegetable soup dumpling
FARÇON   fried sausage and vegetable cake

FARINE   flour
FARINE COMPLÈTE   wholewheat flour
FARINE D'AVOINE   oatmeal
FARINE DE BLÉ   wheat flour
FARINE DE SARRASIN   buckwheat
FARINE DE SEIGLE   rye
FASÉOLE   kidney bean
FAUX   mock or false
FAUX CAFÉ   decaffeinated coffee
FAUX-FILET   sirloin steak
FAVOUILLE   small crab
FÈCHE   dried pork liver
FECHUN   stuffed cabbage
FECOUSE   quiche with bacon, onions, cream
FENOUIL   fennel
FENOUIL GRATINÉ   fennel with cheese
FER À CHEVAL   horseshoe shaped bread
FÉRA   salmon type of lake fish
FERMÉ   closed
FERMETURE   closing
FERMETURE ANNUELLE   closed for holidays and
   vacation
FERMIÈRE   local produce
FERMIÈRE, À LA   braised meat with vegetables
FERMIÈRE, POTAGE À LA   soup of shredded vegetables
   and beans
FEU   fire
FEU DE BOIS, AU   cooked over a wood fire
FEUILLANTINE   pastry with sugar
FEUILLE AU LAIT   pastry crust filled with custard
FEUILLE DE CHÊNE   oak leaf lettuce
FEUILLE DE DREUX   cheese like 'brie' wrapped in chest-
   nut leaves
FEUILLES DE BETTERAVE   beet leaves
FEUILLETÉ   pastry leaves or shell
FEUILLETÉ AUX FRAISES   Napoleon-like pastry with
   strawberries

FEUILLETÉE AU ROQUEFORT   roquefort cheese in puff
   pastry
FÉVEROLES   kidney beans
FÈVES   broad beans or fava beans
FICELLE   very thin, crusty loaf of bread
FICELLE NORMANDE   pancake with ham, cheese in a
   cream sauce
FICELLE PICARDE   ham and mushroom pancake
FIGATELLI   spicy pork sausage
FIGUE   fig
FIGUE DE BARBARIE   prickly pear
FILET   boneless cut of meat
FILET DE BOEUF   fillet of beef
FILET DE BOEUF CROÛTÉ   fillet of beef in pastry
FILET DE BOEUF RÔTI   roast fillet of beef
FILET DE PORC   pork fillet
FILET DE VEAU   veal fillet
FILET GRILLÉ   fillet steak
FILET MIGNON DE PORC NORMANDE   pork with
   apples in cider
FILETS D'ANCHOIS   fillets of anchovies
FILETS DE POISSON MORNAY   fish fillets gratinéed
   with cheese
FILETS DE POISSON, SOUFFLÉ DE   fish soufflé on a platter
FILETS DE POISSONS GRATINÉS AU FOUR   fish fillets
   baked with cheese
FILETS DE POISSONS POCHÉS AU VIN BLANC   fish
   poached in wine
FILETS DE SOLE AMANDINE   fillets of sole cooked with
   butter and almonds
FILETS DE SOLE BONNE FEMME   sole with mushroom
   and wine sauce
FILETS DE SOLE CALYPSO   sole rolled up with finely
   ground lobster
FILETS DE SOLE FRITS   fried fillet of sole
FILETS DE SOLE SYLVESTRE   fish poached in wine with
   vegetables

FILETS MIGNONS DE BOEUF   small cuts of beef
FINES CLAIRES   oysters that have been fattened up
FINES HERBES   mixture of herbs; parsley, chives, tarragon
FIXE   set
FLAGEOLET   a small bean usually green in color
FLAGNARDE   fruit-filled cake
FLAMANDE, À LA   with cabbage, carrots, turnips and potatoes
FLAMBÉ   flamed, usually with brandy
FLAMICHE   leek and cream tart
FLAMMEKUECHE   tart with bacon, onions, cream cheese
FLAMMES   fritters
FLAN   sweet or savory custard
FLANCHET DE BOEUF   flank steak
FLANGNARDE   sweet vanilla pudding baked in a dish
FLET   flounder
FLÉTAN   halibut
FLEUR   flower
FLEURONS   puff pastry garnish
FLOCONS DE MAÏS   corn flakes
FLORENTINE   with spinach
FLORENTINE, POTAGE   cream of spinach soup
FLOTTANTE, ÎLE   cake with whipped cream and custard
FLOUTES   potato balls
FLÛTE   a thin roll
FOIE   liver
FOIE AUX RAISINS   chicken liver cooked in wine with grapes
FOIE DE CANARD   preserved duck livers
FOIE DE POULET   chicken liver
FOIE DE VEAU   calf's liver
FOIE DE VEAU À LA MOUTARDE   calf's liver with mustard and herbs
FOIE DE VEAU SAUTÉ   sautéed calf's liver
FOIE DE VOLAILLE   chicken liver

FOIE DE VOLAILLE, POTAGE DE   cream of chicken liver soup

FOIE DE VOLAILLE SAUTÉ MADÈRE   chicken liver sautéed in Madeira wine sauce

FOIE GRAS   goose liver

FOIE GRAS AUX RAISINS   goose liver with grapes

FOIE GRAS EN CROÛTE   ground livers baked in pastry

FONDANT   frosting for cakes, candies

FONDS   cooking stock

FONDS D'ARTICHAUTS   artichoke bottoms

FONDS DE CUISINE   homemade beef and chicken stocks

FONDU   melted

FONDU AU MARC   soft, mild cheese

FONDUE BOURGUIGNONNE   pieces of meat dipped into boiling oil and eaten with various sauces

FONDUE CHINOISE   thin slices of beef dipped into boiling bouillon then eaten with various sauces

FONDUE DE FROMAGE   melted cheese, wine, kirsch into which bread is dipped

FONDUE FORESTIÈRE   sautéed with mushrooms, potatoes and bacon

FONTAINEBLEAU   cheese made of milk curds and cream

FONTANGES   soup of peas with cream

FORESTIÈRE   garnish of wild mushrooms, bacon and potatoes

FORT   concentrate

FOUACE   sweet cake

FOUÉE   bacon and cream flan

FOUETTÉE   whipped

FOUGASSE   crusty, flat, bread made of flour, water, yeast, may be filled with anchovies or onions

FOUR   baked

FOURCHETTE   fork

FOURME DE MONBRISON   firm cheese, column-shaped, with a bitter taste

FRAISE   strawberry

FRAISES DES BOIS   small wild strawberries
FRAISES MARGUERITE   strawberries with kirsch, sherbet and whipped cream
FRAISES MELBA   strawberries with vanilla ice cream, sauce of strawberries or raspberries
FRAISES ROMANOFF   strawberries in orange flavored liqueur and whipped cream
FRAMBOISE   raspberry, also raspberry liqueur
FRANÇAISE, À LA   French style
FRANGIPANE   almond custard filling
FRAPPÉ   a drink served very cold or with ice
FREMGEYE   fresh cream cheese
FREMIS   lightly cooked oysters
FRESSURE   stew of pig's lung
FRETIN   fried sardines
FRIAND   meat patty
FRIAND À LA MARSEILLAISE   pastry shell filled with tunafish
FRIAND ST. FLOUR   sausage meat in pastry
FRIANDISES   petits fours or cookies
FRICADELLES   chopped meat patties, may have onion and potato, added to soups
FRICANDEAU   sliced veal braised with vegetables and wine
FRICASSÉE   meat, poultry or fish braised in wine or butter with cream
FRICASSÉE DE VEAU   veal stew
FRICASSÉE DE VOLAILLE ET D'ÉCREVISSES   chicken and crayfish stewed in cream and wine
FRISÉE   chicory
FRIT   fried
FRITONS   residue obtained by frying pork fat
FRITOT   small, deep fried pieces of beef, lamb, chicken or veal
FRITURE   oil used for deep frying or fried fish
FRITURE DE LA LOIRE   small deep-fried fish, like sardines
FRIVOLE   fritter

FROID   cold
FROMAGE   cheese
FROMAGE À LA CRÈME   cream cheese
FROMAGE AU MARC DE RAISIN   sweet, usually in a
   crust of grape jelly
FROMAGE BLANC   cream cheese
FROMAGE DE BREBIS   ewe's milk cheese
FROMAGE DE CHÈVRE   goat cheese
FROMAGE DE MONSIEUR   cream cheese
FROMAGE DE PORC   jellied pork loaf
FROMAGE DE TÊTE   head cheese, usually pork
FROMAGE DE VACHE   cow's milk cheese
FROMAGE FRAIS   fresh curd cheese
FROMAGE LE ROI   cream cheese
FROMAGE MAIGRE   low-fat cheese
FROMAGE POUR TARTINER   cheese spread
FRUIT   fruit
FRUIT CONFIT   candied fruit or preserved fruit
FRUIT DE LA PASSION   passion fruit
FRUITS CUITS   stewed fruit
FRUITS DE MER   seafood
FRUITS FRAIS   fresh fruit
FRUITS RAFRAÎCHIS   fruit salad
FUMÉ   smoked
FUMÉES, MOULES   smoked mussels
FUMET   fish stock

G

GALABART   black pudding
GALANTINE   boneless meat or poultry stuffed, cooked,
   sliced and served cold
GALETTE   flat round cake
GALETTE DE POMMES DE TERRE   potato pancake
GALETTE LAUSANNOISE   pastry filled with onions and
   cheese
GALETTE LYONNAISE   mashed potatoes and onions

GALICIEN   sponge cake with cream and apricot jam icing
GALOPIN   thick pancake with brown sugar
GAMBAS   large prawns
GANACHE   chocolate whipped cream filling for cake
GARBURE   soup of cabbage, carrots, beans and salt pork
GARDON   variety of carp
GARENNE, LAPIN DE   wild rabbit
GARNI   garnished
GARNITURE   garnish
GASCONNADE   roasted leg of mutton
GASTRONOME   food connoisseur
GASTRONOME, SAUCE   dark sauce made with white wine
GÂTEAU   cake made without yeast
GÂTEAU À LA BASQUAISE   pastry filled with custard or fruit
GÂTEAU À LA PARISIENNE   meringue covered sponge-cake with almond cream
GÂTEAU ALCAZAR   almond and apricot cake
GÂTEAU AU CHOCOLAT   chocolate cake
GÂTEAU AU FROMAGE   cheese tart
GÂTEAU AUX MARRONS   chestnut cake
GÂTEAU AUX NOISETTES   walnut cake
GÂTEAU GLACÉ   cake and ice cream in slices
GÂTEAU GRENOBLOIS   walnut cake
GÂTEAU LUCULLUS   chocolate chestnut cake
GAUDES   corn flour porridge
GAUFRE   waffle
GAUFRETTE   crisp, sweet wafer
GAYETTES   sausage patties with pork liver and bacon
GAZEUX   carbonated
GEBIE   small shellfish
GELÉE DE GROSEILLES   currant jelly
GELÉE DE VIANDE   wine flavored meat jelly
GELINOTTE   prairie chicken or grouse
GENIÈVRE   juniper berry
GÉNOISE   butter spongecake

GÉNOISE, SAUCE   sauce of nuts, cream and mayonnaise
GENTILHOMME   pureed lentil soup
GÉRARDMER   mild cow's milk cheese
GERMINY   garnish of sorrel
GERMINY, POTAGE   sorrel and chicken soup
GÉROMÉ   spicy cheese with a strong smell
GÉSIER   gizzard
GIBELOTTE   fricassee of rabbit in wine
GIBELOTTE DE LAPIN   rabbit stew with wine sauce
GIBIER   game
GIBIER À PLUME   feathered game
GIBIER À POIL   furred game
GIBIER DE SAISON   game in season
GIGORIT   pig's head in red wine
GIGOT   leg or haunch
GIGOT D'AGNEAU   roast leg of lamb
GIGOT D'AGNEAU À LA BOULANGÈRE   leg of lamb
   roasted with fried onions and potatoes
GIGOT D'AGNEAU RÔTI   roast leg of lamb on a spit
GIGOT DE MOUTON   leg of mutton
GIGOT FARCI, RÔTI À LA MOUTARDE   stuffed leg of
   lamb roasted in mustard glaze
GIGUE   haunch or hip of game meats
GIN-TONIQUE   gin and tonic, the mixed drink
GINGEMBRE   ginger
GINI   bitter lemon
GIROFLE   cloves
GIROLLE   wild mushroom, also called chanterelle
GIROLLE À LA PROVENÇALE   sautéed with garlic and
   onions
GÎTE   shin of beef
GIVRÉ, FRUIT   citrus fruit sorbets
GLACE   ice cream
GLACE À LA VANILLE   custard ice cream
GLACE AUX FRAISES   strawberry ice cream
GLACE, BISCUIT   ice cream on spongecake with fruit,
   liqueur or sauce

GLACE DE VIANDE   meat glaze from stock
GLACE NAPOLITAINE   ice cream of different flavors
GLAÇON   ice cube
GNOCCHI   potato and flour dumpling
GOMBO   okra
GORENFLOT   garnish of sausage, potatoes and cabbage
GOUGELHOPF   yeast bread
GOUGÈRE BOURGUIGNONNE   puff pastry shell with
   Swiss cheese
GOUGÈRE PÂTE À CHOU   cheese pastry ring
GOUGNETTE   sweet fritter
GOUJON   sardine-like freshwater fish
GOULASCH   beef stew with onions and paprika
GOULASCH VEAU   veal goulash
GOURMANDISES   sweet meats
GOURMET   connoisseur of fine food and wine
GOUSSE D'AIL   clove of garlic
GOÛTER   afternoon tea
GOÛTER DÎNATOIRE   late lunch or early dinner
GOYÈRE   cheese tart
GRAIN DE CAFÉ   coffee bean
GRAIN DE POIVRE   peppercorn
GRAIN DE RAISIN   grape
GRAINE DE MOUTARDE   mustard seed
GRAISSE   fat
GRAISSE NORMANDE   pork and beef fat used for cooking
GRAISSERONS   crisply fried pieces of duck or goose skin,
   may also refer to potted pork
GRAMOLATE   sherbet
GRAND   great
GRAND CRÈME   large or double espresso with milk
GRAND CRU   wine of exceptional quality
GRAND MARNIER   orange liqueur
GRAND VENEUR   a brown sauce with red currant jelly
GRANDE CRÊPE   large pancake
GRANITE   water ice
GRAS   fatty

GRAS-DOUBLE   baked tripe with onions and wine
GRASSET   cut of beef
GRATIN (AU)   dish with a browned cheese and crusty
   breadcrumb topping over cream sauce
GRATIN D'ÉPINARDS   spinach
GRATIN DAUPHINOIS   scalloped potatoes
GRATIN DE FRUITS DE MER   shellfish
GRATIN DE POMMES DE TERRE SAUCISSON   sausage
   and potato casserole
GRATIN DE QUEUES D'ÉCREVISSES   crayfish
GRATIN LANDAIS   potato, ham and cheese dish
GRATIN SAVOYARD   casserole of potatoes, bouillon,
   cheese and butter
GRATINÉE   soup with cheese and croutons browned in
   the oven to melt cheese
GRATINÉE LYONNAISE   beef consommé
GRATINÉE, SOUPE   onion soup
GRATTONS   crisp fried pork, goose, or duck skin
GRATUIT   free
GRECQUE, À LA   cold vegetables in seasoned oil and
   lemon juice
GRELOT   small white bulb onion
GRENADE   pomegranate
GRENADIN   small veal scallop
GRENADINS DE BOEUF   beef cooked with vegetables,
   wine, onions and mushrooms
GRENOUILLE   frog
GRENOUILLE BRESSANE   frog's legs in cream sauce
GRENOUILLE, CUISSES DE   frog's legs
GRENOUILLE, POTAGE DE   frogs' leg soup
GRENOUILLE PROVENÇALE   fried frogs' legs
GRIGNAUDES   fried pieces of pork
GRILLADE   grilled meat
GRILLADE AU FENOUIL   grilled with fennel, usually fish
GRILLÉ   grilled
GRILLETTES   bits of fat grilled till crispy
GRIOTTES   red, sour cherries

GRIS DE LILLE   soft cheese, very spicy

GRIVE   thrush

GRONDIN   ocean fish used in stews and bouillabaisse

GROS   oversized or large

GROS SEL   course salt

GROSEILLE   currant

GROSEILLE À MAQUEREAU   gooseberry

GROSEILLE BLANCHE   white currant

GROSEILLE ROUGE   red currant

GRUAU   very fine flour

GRUYÈRE   hard, mild Swiss cheese

GRUYÈRE DE BEAUFORT   salty and fruity cow's milk
   cheese

GRUYÈRE DE COMTÉ   firm sharp tasting cows' milk
   cheese

GRYPHÉE   Portuguese oyster

GUEUZELAMBIC   Flemish bitter beer

GUIGNE   cherry

GUILLARET   sweet pastry

GUITARE   sea skate

GYMNÈTRE   Mediterranean cod fish

H

HACHIS   minced or chopped meat or fish, like hash

HACHIS DE BOEUF   minced beef

HACHIS PARMENTIER   shepherd's pie of minced meat
   in sauce

HACHUA   ham stewed with peppers and onions

HARENG   herring

HARENG BLANC   salt herring

HARENG FRAIS   fresh herring

HARENG FUMÉ   smoked herring

HARENG LUCAS   smoked herring in mustard mayonnaise sauce

HARENG ROULÉ   marinated herring

HARENG SALÉ   salted kippered herring
HARENG SAUR   red herring
HARICOT   bean
HARICOT BEURRE   butter bean
HARICOT BLANC   white lima bean
HARICOT D'ESPAGNE   runner bean
HARICOT DE MOUTON   stew, with mutton and white beans
HARICOT DE LIMA   lima bean
HARICOT MANGE-TOUT   runner beans
HARICOT ROUGE   red kidney bean
HARICOT VERT   french green bean
HARICOTS VERTS À LA LYONNAISE   green beans cooked with onions
HARICOTS VERTS À LA PROVENÇALE   french beans with tomato
HARICOTS VERTS AU NATUREL   green string beans, blanched and buttered
HÂTELETTE   cooked on a skewer
HAUTE   high
HAUTE CUISINE   classic French cooking
HÉNON   cockle, like small sea clam
HÉRISSON   hedgehog
HIRONDELLE   swallow
HOCHEPOT   thick stew, usually oxtail
HOLLANDAISE   egg yolks and lemon in cream with butter added
HOMARD   lobster
HOMARD À L'AMÉRICAINE   lobster pieces sautéed in butter, flamed with cognac, then simmered in wine and vegetables
HOMARD À LA CHARENTAISE   lobster in cream sauce with cognac and grape juice
HOMARD À LA CRÈME   lobster with cream sauce
HOMARD À LA PARISIENNE   lobster pieces served with mixed vegetables in the shell

HOMARD À LA SUÉDOISE   baked lobster meat, anchovies and cream sauce

HOMARD CALVAISE   lobster in spicy tomato sauce

HOMARD CARDINAL   lobster flamed in brandy

HOMARD GRATINÉ FROMAGE   lobster steamed in wine and gratinéed

HOMARD NEWBURG   lobster sautéed in Madeira wine and cream sauce

HOMARD THERMIDOR   lobster simmered in wine, butter, mushrooms; flamed and gratinéed with cheese

HONGROISE, À L'   with paprika and cream

HORS-D'OEUVRE   first course

HORS-D'OEUVRE ASSORTIS   mixed hors d'oeuvres

HORS-D'OEUVRE RICHES   deluxe appetizers

HORS-D'OEUVRE VARIÉS   salami and cold meats

HÔTE   guest or host

HÔTELIÈRE   with parsley butter

HOUBLON   hops

HOUX   holly

HUILE   cooking oil

HUILE D'AMANDE   almond oil

HUILE D'ARACHIDE   peanut oil

HUILE D'OLIVE   olive oil

HUILE DE MAÏS   corn oil

HUILE DE NOIX   walnut oil

HUILE DE SOJA   soya bean oil

HUILE DE TOURNESOL   sunflower oil

HUÎTRE   oyster

HUÎTRE DE BELON   flat, pinkish oyster

HUÎTRE FINE CLAIRE   like bluepoint oyster

HUÎTRE PORTUGAISE   small oyster

HUÎTRIER   marsh bird

HURE DE PORC   pig's head in jelly

HURE DE SAUMON   pâté prepared with salmon

HURE MARCASSIN   a head cheese prepared from boar

HYPOCRAS   spiced red wine

I

IGNAME   yam (tropical root vegetable)

ÎLE FLOTTANTE   spongecake sprinkled with kirsch, maraschinos, currants, almonds and covered with crème anglaise

IMPÉRATRICE (RIZ À L')   rice pudding dessert with candied fruit

IMPÉRIAL   cream of celery soup

INDIENNE, POTAGE À L'   cream soup with chicken, rice and curry

INDIENNE, SAUCE À L'   with rice or curry

INFUSION   herb tea

IRLANDAISE, À L'   served with potatoes

ISSUE DE SECOURS   emergency exit

IZARRA   liqueur similar to Chartreuse

J

JACQUE   apple pancake

JAMBON   ham

JAMBON À LA BAYONNAISE   ham with sausage, mushrooms, tomatoes and rice

JAMBON À LA CRÈME   ham in cream sauce

JAMBON AU CIDRE   ham cooked in cider

JAMBON AURORE   cooked ham in a butter, cream, tomato sauce

JAMBON BLANC   boiled ham

JAMBON BRAISÉ   braised ham in sherry wine

JAMBON CRU   raw cured ham

JAMBON CUIT   cooked ham

JAMBON D'AUVERGNE   raw, dried, salt cured smoked ham

JAMBON D'OIE   breast of smoked goose like ham in taste

JAMBON D'YORK   smoked English ham, often poached

JAMBON DE BAYONNE   cured ham in thin slices

JAMBON DE BOURGOGNE   cold cooked ham in gelatin
JAMBON DE CAMPAGNE   country smoked ham
JAMBON DE CANARD   smoked breast of duck, like ham
   in taste
JAMBON DE MONTAGNE   country smoked ham
   mountain style
JAMBON DE PARIS   cooked ham
JAMBON DE PARME   smoked ham eaten raw in paper-
   thin slices, prosciutto ham
JAMBON DE WESTPHALIE   German Westphalian ham,
   raw-cured and smoked
JAMBON DU PAYS   country ham, usually salt cured
JAMBON EN CROÛTE   ham in pastry
JAMBON FOIN   ham simmered in water with herbs
JAMBON FROID   cold ham
JAMBON FUMÉ   smoked ham
JAMBON, L'OS DE   ham bone
JAMBON MADÈRE   ham prepared with a Madeira wine
JAMBON PERSILLÉ   cold preserved ham in gelatin
JAMBON POCHÉ   ham poached in stock
JAMBON SALÉ   salt cured ham
JAMBON SAUPIQUET   ham in wine and cream sauce
JAMBON SEC   dried ham
JAMBONNEAU   cured ham shank
JAMBONNETTE   boned and stuffed knuckle of ham
JARDINIÈRE   garnish of fresh cooked vegetables
JARNAC   sponge cake with jam and cognac
JARRET   knuckle
JARRET DE BOEUF EN DAUBE   shin of beef stewed with
   wine in a casserole
JARRET DE PORC SALÉ   salted shin of pork
JARRET DE VEAU   veal shin
JARRET DE VEAU AU CITRON   stewed knuckle of veal
   with lemon
JAUNE D'OEUF   egg yolk
JEREZ   Spanish sherry
JÉSUITE   flaky pastry with almond paste

JÉSUS   sausage
JÉSUS DE MORTEAU   smoked sausage
JETONS   tokens for the telephone
JEUNE   young
JOURNEAUX   chicken liver sauce
JUBILÉ, POTAGE   pea soup with vegetables
JUIF   Jewish style
JULIENNE   slivered vegetables or meat
JULIENNE, BOUILLON   bouillon with vegetables
JULIENNE, POTAGE   vegetable soup
JUS   juice
JUS DE CITRON   lemon juice
JUS DE FRUITS   fruit juice
JUS DE POMMES   apple juice
JUS DE TOMATE   tomato juice

K

KAFFEKRANTZ   raisin cake
KAKI   persimmon
KARI   curry
KASSLER   rolled pork fillet
KEBAB   meat cooked on a skewer
KIG HA FARS   slow cooked meat and vegetable casserole
KIPPER   smoked herring
KIR   white wine mixed with black currant liqueur
KIR ROYAL   champagne mixed with black currant
    liqueur
KIRSCH   cherry liqueur
KISSEL   dessert of mixed berries with cream cheese
KNACKWURST   sausage
KNEPFLE   dumpling
KOKEBOTEROM   raisin muffin
KOUGLOF   sweet, round Alsatian yeast cake, with
    almonds and raisins
KOUIGN AMANN   puff pastry cake
KUGELHOPF   brioche cake with almonds and raisins

KUMMEL   caraway seed liqueur
KUMQUAT   miniature orange

L

LAIT   milk
LAIT BARRATTÉ   buttermilk
LAIT DEMI-ÉCRÉMÉ   semi skimmed milk
LAIT ÉCRÉMÉ   skimmed milk
LAIT RIBOT   a yoghurt drink
LAIT STÉRILISÉ   long life milk
LAITAGE   dairy product
LAITANCE   fish roe milt, fish eggs
LAITANCE SABOT   baked potatoes stuffed with herring
    roe
LAITERIE   dairy shop or creamery
LAITUE   lettuce
LAITUE BRAISÉE   braised lettuce
LAITUE PAYSANNE   lettuce cooked with ham, onions
    and carrots
LAMBALLE   soup of pureed peas thickened with tapioca
LAMBEAU   scrap
LAME   very thin slice
LAMPROIE   lamprey, an eel shaped fish
LAMPROIE À LA BORDELAISE   eel in red wine
LANDAISE   cooked in garlic and onions with goose fat
LANGOUSTE   lobster
LANGOUSTE À LA DIABLE   spicy baked lobster
LANGOUSTE SÉTOISE   lobster in spicy tomato sauce
    with brandy
LANGOUSTE WINTERTHUR   lobster with shrimp and
    mushroom, gratinéed
LANGOUSTINE   large prawn
LANGUE   tongue
LANGUE À L'ÉCARLATE   salted tongue
LANGUE D'AGNEAU BRAISÉE AUX PETITS POIS
    braised lamb tongue

LANGUE DE BOEUF   ox tongue
LANGUE DE BOEUF BRAISÉE AU MADÈRE   beef tongue braised in Madeira sauce
LANGUE DE VEAU   calf's tongue
LANGUE FOURRÉE   stuffed tongue
LANGUEDOCIENNE   tomatoes and wild mushrooms
LANGUEDOCIENNE, GRATIN À LA   baked eggplant with tomatoes, breadcrumbs and garlic
LANGUEDOCIENNE, PÂTÉ DE PIGEON À LA   pigeon pie with mushrooms and chicken livers
LANGUIER   smoked pork tongue
LAPEREAU   young rabbit
LAPIN   rabbit
LAPIN À LA HAVRAISE   roast rabbit with bacon in cream sauce
LAPIN DE GARENNE   wild rabbit
LARD   bacon
LARD DE POITRINE FUMÉ   smoked bacon slab
LARDONS   cubes of fried bacon
LASAGNE   baked pasta and cheese with meat sauce
LAURIER   bay leaves
LAVARET   fish related to the salmon
LEBERKNEPFEN   calf's liver dumplings
LÈCHE   thin slice of bread or meat
LÉGUME   vegetable
LÉGUME À LA GRECQUE   marinated vegetables, Greek style
LÉGUMES, POTAGE DE   vegetable soup
LENTILLE   lentil
LENTILLES (POTAGE DE)   lentil soup
LEWERKNOPFLES   liver dumplings
LIBRE   free
LIÉGEOIS   soft ice cream dessert
LIÉGEOISE   made with juniper berries and gin
LIERWECKE   raisin bun
LIEU JAUNE   pollack, a small saltwater fish
LIÈVRE   hare

LIÈVRE À LA PIRON   hare marinated and roasted in a peppery cream sauce

LIÈVRE À LA ROYALE   dish of hare, ground livers, wine and truffles

LIMACE   small snail

LIMANDE   fish similar to sole

LIMANDE, SOLE   lemon sole

LIMON   lime

LIMONADE   fizzy lemonade

LIMOUSINE, À LA   red cabbage, chestnuts and mushrooms

LINGUE   cod fish

LISETTE   small mackerel

LIVAROT   soft paste cheese

LIVORNAISE (SAUCE)   olive oil, egg yolks and anchovy paste

LONGCHAMP   peas, sorrel and chervil soup

LONGE   loin

LONGE DE VEAU   loin of veal

LONGUET   breadstick

LONGUEVILLE   soup with leeks and peas

LORRAINE, À LA   braised in wine

LOTTE   monkfish

LOU MAGRET   breast of fattened duck

LOUBIA   dried kidney beans

LOUBINE   gray mullet fish

LOUKINKA   garlic sausage

LOUP   bass fish

LOUP AU FENOUIL   sea bass flambéed in brandy

LOUP DE MER   Mediterranean fish, similar to striped bass

LYONNAISE, À LA   garnished with onions; in the style of Lyons

M

MACARON   macaroon

MACÉDOINE DE FRUITS   diced mixed fruit or vegetables

MACÉDOINE DE LÉGUMES   salad of cooked vegetables in mayonnaise

MÂCHE   like a butter lettuce

MADELEINES   small tea cakes

MAGISTÈRE   meat and vegetable soup

MAGNUM   double size champagne bottle

MAGRET DE CANARD   breast of duck, grilled rare

MAIGRE   lean, a meatless preparation

MAÏS   corn

MAISON   restaurant or house

MAÎTRE DE CHAI   master in charge of wine making

MAMIROLLE   soft, strong cheese

MANDARIN   bitter, orange flavored drink

MANDARINE   tangerine

MANGE   eat

MANGE-TOUT   a green runner bean, a snow pea

MANGUE   mango

MANQUE   sponge cake with crystallized fruit

MAQUEREAU   mackerel

MAQUEREAU À LA BOULONNAISE   poached mackerel with mussels

MAQUEREAU AU VIN BLANC   mackerel poached in white wine

MAQUEREAU EN PAPILLOTE   mackerel baked in paper

MAQUEREAU GRILLÉ   grilled mackerel

MAQUEREAU MARINÉ   pickled or marinated mackerel

MARC   type of brandy

MARC DE BOURGOGNE   brandy distilled from pressed grape skins and seeds

MARCASSIN   young wild boar

MARCASSIN À L'ARDENNAISE   roasted wild boar in red wine sauce

MARCASSIN FARCI AU SAUCISSON   boar stuffed with sausage

MARCHAND DE VIN   dark brown sauce made with meat and wine

MARENNES   flat shelled, green tinged plate oysters

MARGARINE   margarine
MARGUERY, SAUCE   white wine and seafood sauce
MARIGNAN   cake with liqueur, apricot jam and meringue
MARIGNY   pea soup with French beans and peas
MARINÉ   marinated
MARINIÈRE   seafood in white wine and spices
MARINIÈRE MOULES   mussels in white wine with
   onions, shallots, butter and herbs
MARJOLAINE   marjoram, an herb
MARLY   rum or kirsch flavored cake with strawberries
   and cream
MARMITE   a rich meat soup
MARMITE DIEPPOISE   fish stewed in white wine and
   cream
MAROILLES   strong, semi-hard cheese
MARQUISE AU CHOCOLAT   spongecake filled and
   covered with chocolate cream
MARRON   large chestnut
MARRON GLACÉ   candied chestnut
MASSEPAIN   almond paste
MATAFAN   thick potato pancake
MATELOTE   fish stew
MATELOTE CANOTIÈRE   carp and eel stew
MATELOTE D'ANGUILLE   eel and fish stew
MATELOTE, SAUCE   made with wine, garlic and shallots
MAUVIETTE   wild meadowlark or skylark game birds
MAYONNAISE   dressing of egg yolks, vinegar or lemon
   juice
MAYONNAISE, CRABE À LA   cold crab appetizer
MAYONNAISE, POISSON À LA   fish with mayonnaise
MAYORQUINA   cabbage and tomato soup with onions
   and leeks
MAZARIN   sponge cake filled with crystallized fruit
MÉDAILLON   a small, circular cut of meat or poultry
MÉDAILLON DE VEAU   miniature veal steak
MEHLSUPPE   leek and onion soup
MÉLANGE   mixture

MELON   melon
MELON À L'ITALIENNE   melon wrapped in thin slices of raw-cured ham
MELON D'EAU   watermelon
MELON DE CAVAILLON   small melon, like canteloupe
MELON FRAPPÉ   melon filled with sherbet
MELON GLACÉ   iced melon
MELON GLACÉ AU PORTO   iced melon pieces in port wine
MELON SUCRIN   honeydew melon
MELON SURPRISE   melon filled with fruit and liqueur
MÉNAGÈRE   a preparation of onions, potatoes and carrots
MENON   roast goat
MENTHE   sweet, green mint-flavored syrup
MENTHE POIVRÉE   peppermint
MENU GASTRONOMIQUE   expensive menu for gourmets
MENU PRIX FIXE   set price meal
MERCI   thank you
MERGUEZ   small spicy sausage
MERINGUE   stiffly beaten egg whites
MERINGUE AUX NOISETTES   meringue with toasted nuts
MERINGUE GLACÉE   beaten egg whites baked and cooled, and served with ice cream
MERINGUE ITALIENNE   sugar-syrup meringue mixture
MERINGUETTES   baked finger lengths of stiffly beaten egg whites
MERLAN   whiting
MERLE   blackbird pâté
MERLU   dried cod fish
MERLUCHE   dried cod fish
MERVEILLE   small cake cooked in oven or deep fried with brandy or rum
MERVEILLES À LA CHARENTAISE   small cakes with cognac

MESCLUN   salad of mixed lettuces

MESSIEURS   gentlemen

METURE   corn fritter

MEUNIÈRE   fish seasoned, floured, fried in butter

MEURETTE   red wine sauce

MEURETTE, VOLAILLE EN   chicken stew with red wine,
    onions, as coq au vin

MICHE   round loaf of bread

MIEL   honey

MIGNARDISE   petit-four

MIJOT   soup of red wine and bread

MIJOTER   simmer

MILANAIS   spongecake with liqueur, apricot jam and
    aniseed icing

MILANAISE, À LA   vegetable, ham and sausage soup
    with grated cheese

MILLASSOU   sweet corn custard

MILLE-FEUILLE   Napoleon pastry

MILLÉSIME   year of the wine

MILLIASSON   sweet corn flour pastry

MIMOLETTE   tangy, semi-hard cheese similar to Edam

MIMOSA   garnish of chopped, hard-boiled egg yolks

MINÉRALE, EAU   mineral water

MIQUE SARLADAISE   soup with dumpling made with
    corn flour and pork fat

MIRABEAU   anchovies, garlic, lemon juice

MIRABELLE   brandy from yellow plums

MIRABELLES   small yellow-green plums

MIREPOIX   cubes of carrots and onions or mixed
    vegetables

MIRLITONS   tart with almond-cream filling

MIROTON   stew of meats flavored with onions

MIROTON, BOEUF   sliced boiled beef in onion and sour
    pickle sauce sprinkled with cheese

MIS EN BOUTEILLES AU CHÂTEAU   bottled at the
    château

MODE   in the fashion or style

MOELLE   beef bone marrow

MOELLEUX   mellow sweet wines

MOKA   coffee, or coffee flavored dish

MOKATINE   coffee flavored petit-four

MONACO   with a green pea and caper sauce

MONGLE   pea and tomato soup

MONT BLANC   dessert of mashed chestnuts and whipped cream

MONT D'OR   soft, mild cheese with a delicate taste

MONT DES CATS, ABBAYE DE   soft, mild cheese

MONTAGNARDE   vegetable soup with grated cheese

MONTÉ-CRISTO   flan with almond filling

MONTRACHET   goat cheese which is wrapped in chestnut leaves

MORBIER   firm cheese with black streak and fruity taste

MORILLE   wild morel mushroom, dark brown and conical shaped

MORNAY   thick, milk based sauce with flour, butter, egg yolks and cheese

MORTADELLE   large sausage

MORUE   salted or dried codfish

MORUE AUX ÉPINARDS   codfish prepared with spinach

MORUE PROVENÇALE   salt cod with garlic and onion sauce

MORUE SALÉE   salt cod

MOSTELE   small Mediterranean fish

MOUCLADE   creamy mussel stew with curry

MOULE   mussel

MOULES À LA POULETTE   mussels in white sauce with mushrooms

MOULES D'ESPAGNE   large raw mussels

MOULES FARCIES   stuffed mussels

MOULES MARINIÈRE   boiled mussels in white wine with shallots and parsley

MOULES NORMANDE   mussels in wine and cream sauce

MOURTAYROL   ham, chicken, beef, and vegetable soup

MOUSSAKA   a Greek lamb and eggplant dish

MOUSSE   beaten egg whites or whipped cream; meat, poultry or fish finely ground and served in a mold

MOUSSE AU CHOCOLAT   chocolate, egg yolks, sugar, beaten to mousse consistency

MOUSSE DE FOIE GRAS   ground goose livers with cream and whipped with truffles

MOUSSE DE VOLAILLE EN GELÉE   cold chicken, whipped, then served with aspic

MOUSSE GLACÉE AUX FRAISES   strawberry sherbet whipped until frothy

MOUSSELINE   ground fish beaten with egg white and cream, cooked in patties

MOUSSELINE DE POISSON MARÉCHALE   fish cakes with vinegar and wine, butter and shallot sauce

MOUSSELINE, SAUCE   Hollandaise sauce enriched with whipped cream

MOUSSERON   delicate wild spring mushroom

MOUSSERON À LA CRÈME   mushroom in cream sauce

MOUSSEUX   sparkling or frothy

MOUTARDE   mustard

MOUTON   mutton

MOUTON AUX PISTACHES   mutton braised in wine with garlic, vegetables and pistachio nuts

MULET   gray mullet fish

MULLIGATAWNY   curry soup with onions and potatoes

MUNSTER   soft cheese

MÛRE   blackberry

MÛRE SAUVAGE   wild blackberry

MUSCADE   nutmeg

MUSCADELLE   pear

MUSCADET   white wine

MUSCAT   dessert wine

MUSEAU DE PORC   vinegared pork muzzle or snout

MYE   clam

MYRTILLE   blueberry-like berry

MYSTÈRE   dessert of meringue, ice cream and chocolate sauce

N

NAGE, À LA   cooked and served in bouillon poaching liquid

NANTAIS   almond biscuit

NAPOLITAIN   almond cake with fruit jam

NAPOLITAINE   vanilla, strawberry and chocolate ice cream, sliced

NAPPE   tablecloth

NATUREL, AU   in a natural state

NAVARIN   lamb or mutton stew with potatoes and onions

NAVARIN AUX POMMES   mutton stew with potatoes and tomatoes

NAVARIN D'AGNEAU   brown lamb stew

NAVARIN DE MOUTON   roasted mutton stew with consommé, onions, cloves, potatoes

NAVARIN PRINTANIER   lamb stew with carrots, onions, potatoes, turnips, green peas and beans

NAVET   turnip

NAVET À LA CHAMPENOISE   turnip and onion casserole

NAVET GLACÉ   glazed turnip

NÈGRE EN CHEMISE   chocolate dessert with whipped cream

NEIGE, CITRON À LA   lemon flavored shaved ice

NELUSKO   petit four with brandied cherries and red currant jam

NÉROLI   oil extracted from the flowers of orange trees

NESSELRODE   dessert or sauce containing fruits, chestnuts and whipped cream

NEWBURG   lobster prepared with Madeira, egg yolks and cream

NEWBURG, SAUCE   creamy sauce made with egg yolks, cream, sherry, and pieces of lobster

NIÇOISE, SALADE   salad of vegetables, onions, anchovies, tunafish, artichokes and beans

NIÇOISE, À LA   refers to dishes with onions, garlic, olive oil, tomatoes, anchovies

NIVERNAISE, À LA   garnish of carrots, onions, potatoes

NOILLY PRAT   vermouth

NOISETTE   hazelnut, also small round piece, as in potato, generally size of a hazelnut, lightly browned in butter

NOISETTE D'AGNEAU   lamb cutlet from the fillet

NOISETTE D'AGNEAU CLAMART   lamb, artichoke hearts and peas

NOISETTINE NONNETTE   two layers of gingerbread pastry with hazelnut cream

NOIX   nuts in general, but also walnuts

NOIX DE BRÉSIL   Brazil nuts

NOIX DE COCO   coconut

NOIX DE MUSCADE   nutmeg

NOIX DE VEAU   center cut of veal

NORMANDE, À LA   fish or meat cooked with apple cider; apple dessert with cream

NORMANDE, SAUCE   fish cream sauce with mushrooms, wine or cider

NOS SPECIALITÉS   our specialties

NOS VINS   our wines

NOUGAT   sweet candy made of almonds and nougat

NOUGAT GLACÉ   burnt almond ice cream

NOUGATINE   vanilla spongecake with praline cream and chocolate icing

NOUILLES   noodles

NOUILLES AU FROMAGE   noodles with cheese

NOUZILLARDS AU LAIT   chestnut and milk soup

O

OCCUPÉ   engaged

OEUF   eggs, also see omelettes

OEUF À L'AGENAISE   baked egg with fried eggplant and onion

OEUF À L'AUTRICHIENNE   poached egg with cabbage and sausages

OEUF À L'HONGROISE   hard egg with onions and mayonnaise

OEUF À LA BRETONNE   egg stuffed with onions, mushrooms and leeks

OEUF À LA DIABLE   deviled egg

OEUF À LA FLORENTINE   egg served with spinach

OEUF À LA LORRAINE   egg baked with cheese and bacon

OEUF À LA MAZARINE   egg custard with tomato sauce

OEUF À LA MÉNAGÈRE   fried egg on macaroni with tomato sauce

OEUF À LA NEIGE   egg white sweetened and poached in milk and vanilla custard

OEUF À LA PARISIENNE   baked egg, mushrooms and ground chicken

OEUF À LA PÉRIGOURDINE   egg baked with ground goose liver

OEUF À LA RUSSE   hard egg yolk mixed with mayonnaise and herbs

OEUF AMIRAL   egg mixed with pieces of lobster

OEUF ARGENTEUIL   scrambled egg with asparagus tips

OEUF AU BEURRE NOIR   egg with brown butter

OEUF AU JAMBON   ham and egg

OEUF AU LARD   egg with bacon

OEUF AUX AUBERGINES FRITES   egg with fried eggplant

OEUF BELLEVILLOISE   baked egg in a cream sauce with sausage

OEUF BÉNÉDICTINE   poached egg with ham and hollandaise sauce

OEUF BERCY   baked egg with sausage and tomato sauce

OEUF BROUILLÉ   scrambled egg

OEUF CHASSEUR   scrambled egg with chicken livers

OEUF COCOTTE   egg baked in custard cups with cream

OEUF COCOTTE À LA REINE AUX TOMATES   baked
  egg with macaroni, tomatoes and béchamel sauce
OEUF COQUE   boiled egg
OEUF DE POISSON   egg with fish roe
OEUF DUR   hard-boiled egg
OEUF DUR À LA TRIPE   hard-boiled egg in onion sauce
OEUF EN GELÉE   poached egg in aspic or wine flavored
  jelly
OEUF EN MEURETTE   poached egg in red wine sauce
OEUF FARCI   stuffed egg
OEUF FRIT   fried egg
OEUF GRAND-DUC   poached egg in mornay sauce with
  asparagus tips
OEUF LUCULLUS   poached egg on artichoke heart in
  cream sauce with foie gras
OEUF MIRETTE   tart with a poached egg yolk and
  chicken in a cream sauce
OEUF MOLLET   five-minute boiled egg
OEUF PASCAL   egg baked in mustard and cream sauce
OEUF POCHÉ   poached egg
OEUF POCHÉ EN MEURETTE   poached egg in red wine
  sauce
OEUF POCHÉ SOUFFLÉ À LA FLORENTINE   soufflé of
  poached egg on creamed spinach
OEUF POÊLÉ   sunny-side-up fried egg
OEUF ROSSINI   egg, truffles and Madeira wine
OEUF SUR CANAPÉ   egg, ham and cheese on bread
OEUFS À L'AGENAISE   baked eggs with fried eggplant
  and onion
OIE   goose
OIE BRAISÉE AUX PRUNEAUX   braised goose with
  prune and liver stuffing
OIE EN DAUBE   goose, stewed with wine
OIE RÔTIE AUX PRUNEAUX   roast goose with prune stuffing
OIGNON   onion
OIGNONS BLANCS GLACÉS   glazed white onions
OISEAU   bird

OISEAUX SANS TÊTES   pieces of meat rolled up and
stuffed with varying ingredients

OISON   a young goose

OLIVES FARCIES NOIRES   stuffed black olives

OLIVES FARCIES VERTES   stuffed green olives

OLIVES NOIRES   black olives

OLIVES VERTES   green olives

OMBLE   lake trout, like salmon

OMBLE-CHEVALIER   felchen from Lake Constance

OMELETTE   eggs usually whipped with other ingredients,
also see oeufs

OMELETTE À L'ALGÉRIENNE   omelette with eggplant
and artichokes

OMELETTE À L'ESPAGNOLE   omelette with tomato
sauce, onions, Spanish omelette

OMELETTE À L'OIGNON   omelette with sautéed
chopped onions

OMELETTE À LA BASQUAISE   omelette with green
peppers, tomatoes and ham

OMELETTE AU CHOIX   omelette with filling of your choice

OMELETTE AU FOIE DE VOLAILLE   omelette with
chicken liver

OMELETTE AU FROMAGE   omelette with cheese

OMELETTE AU FROMAGE OU JAMBON   omelette with
cheese or ham

OMELETTE AU GRUYÈRE   omelette with grated Swiss
cheese

OMELETTE AUX CROÛTONS   omelette with fried bread

OMELETTE AUX ÉPINARDS   omelette with spinach

OMELETTE AUX FINES HERBES   omelette with herbs

OMELETTE AUX FRUITS DE MER   omelette with seafood

OMELETTE AUX POINTES D'ASPERGES   omelette with
asparagus

OMELETTE AUX TOMATES   omelette with tomato

OMELETTE AUX TRUFFES   omelette with truffles

OMELETTE BONNE FEMME   omelette with onions and
chopped bacon

OMELETTE CÉLESTINE   omelette with mushrooms
OMELETTE CLAMART   omelette with fresh peas and green onions
OMELETTE DE CREVETTES   omelette with shrimp
OMELETTE FLAMBÉE AU RHUM   dessert omelet with flaming rum
OMELETTE GRATINÉE AUX CHAMPIGNONS   omelette with mushroom and cheese sauce
OMELETTE LIMOUSINE   omelette with fried potatoes and ham
OMELETTE LYONNAISE   omelette with onions
OMELETTE MAINTENON   omelette with chicken and mushrooms in white onion sauce with browned cheese
OMELETTE NATURE   whipped eggs, pancake style
OMELETTE NIÇOISE   omelette with tomato and anchovies
OMELETTE NORMANDE   omelette with mushrooms and shrimps
OMELETTE NORVÉGIENNE   ice cream with meringue topping baked, like Baked Alaska
OMELETTE PARISIENNE   omelette with onion, mushroom and sausages
OMELETTE PARMENTIER   omelet with boiled potatoes
OMELETTE PROVENÇALE   omelette with garlic, tomatoes and onions
OMELETTE SAVOYARDE   omelette with leeks, potatoes and cheese
OMELETTE SOUFFLÉE À LA LIQUEUR   liqueur flavored soufflé
OMELETTE SURPRISE   meringue and ice cream, browned on top, like Baked Alaska
ORANGE   orange
ORANGE GIVRÉE   orange ice or sherbet in an orange shell
ORANGE PRESSÉ   fresh squeezed orange juice served with a carafe of water and sugar for sweetening
ORANGEADE   orange flavored water
OREILLES DE PORC   cooked pig's ears, served grilled with a coating of egg and bread crumbs

ORGE   barley
ORONGES   wild mushroom
ORTOLAN   small game bird like a finch
OS   bone
OS À LA MOELLE   marrow bone
OSEILLE   sorrel, herb
OUILAT   onion soup with beans, leeks and cheese
OUILLADE   soup of cabbage and beans
OULADE   stew made from potatoes, cabbage, sausage
   and pork
OURSIN   sea urchin
OUVERT   open
OYONNADE   goose stewed in wine

P

PACARET   made with sherry
PAGRE   pompano type fish in bream family
PAILLARDE, VEAU   grilled boneless veal steak or cutlet
PAILLES   straws
PAILLETÉ, OIGNON   fried onion rings
PAILLETTES   cheese straws made with puff pastry
PAIN   bread
PAIN AUX RAISINS   rye or wheat bread filled with
   raisins
PAIN AZYME   unleavened bread
PAIN BIS   brown bread
PAIN COMPLET   whole-grain bread
PAIN DE BROCHET D'ANGOULÊME   fish loaf of pike
PAIN DE CAMPAGNE   country loaf
PAIN DE FROMENT   wheat bread
PAIN DE GÊNES   almond cake
PAIN DE MIE   sandwich bread
PAIN DE NOIX and PAIN DE NOISETTES   rye or wheat
   bread with walnuts or hazelnuts
PAIN D'ÉPICE   gingerbread or spice cake
PAIN DE POISSON   loaf of ground fish

PAIN DE SEIGLE   bread made from rye flour and some wheat flour

PAIN DE SON   diet bread containing 20% bran

PAIN ET COUVERT COMPRIS or NON-COMPRIS   bread and table setting included or not included

PAIN FANTAISIE   odd shaped bread

PAIN GRILLÉ   toast

PAIN POLKA   large country loaf bread

PAIN RÔTI   toast

PAIN SANS SEL   salt free bread

PAIN VIENNOIS   baguette shaped white bread

PALERON   shoulder of beef

PALERON DE BOEUF   chuck or pot roast

PALISSADE DE MARRONS   molded chestnut and chocolate dessert

PALMIER   palm leaf shaped cookie made of sugared puff pastry

PALOMBE   wood or wild pigeon

PALOURDE   medium size clam

PAMPLEMOUSSE   grapefruit

PAMPLEMOUSSE PRESSÉ   grapefruit juice served with water and sugar for sweetening

PAN BAGNA   roll with tomatoes, anchovies, onions in oil

PANACHÉ   mixed

PANAIS   parsnip

PANÉ   prepared with breadcrumbs

PANNEQUET   pancake

PANTIN   pastry filled with ground pork

PANURE   coating of breadcrumbs

PAPAYE   papaya fruit

PAPILLOTE, EN   cooked in parchment paper or foil envelope

PAPRICA   paprika

PARFAIT   a dessert of ice cream, whipped cream and fruits

PARFUMS DIVERS   different flavors

PARIS-BREST   cream-puff pastry ring with whipped cream filling

PARISIENNE, À LA   varied vegetable garnish including potato balls fried and tossed in a meat glaze
PARMENTIER   dish with potatoes
PARMENTIER, POTAGE   potato soup
PARMESANÉ   prepared with parmesan cheese
PASSE-PIERRE   edible seaweed
PASTA FROLLA   sweet pastry made with kirsch
PASTÈQUE   watermelon
PASTILLE   hard candy of flavored sugar
PASTIS   anise flavored alcohol like Pernod and Ricard
PASTIS GÉNOISE   spongecake with brandy flavoring
PASTIS LANDAISE   prune filled pastry
PATATE   sweet potato
PÂTÉ   minced meat molded, spiced, baked in pastry, served in slices hot or cold
PÂTE À CHOUX   cream puff pastry
PÂTÉ ARDENNAIS   pork and seasonings in pastry
PÂTE BRISÉE   pastry used for pies and tarts
PÂTÉ CHARTRES   partridge in pastry
PÂTÉ CHAUD   small hot patty filled with meat, fish or grated cheese
PÂTÉ CHAUD AU SAUMON   salmon pie
PÂTÉ D'AMANDES   almond paste
PÂTÉ D'ANGUILLE   eel pâté
PÂTÉ D'OIE   goose pâté
PÂTÉ DE BÉCASSE   woodcock pâté
PÂTÉ DE BIFTECK   beefsteak pie
PÂTÉ DE CAMPAGNE   pork pâté
PÂTÉ DE CANARD   duck pâté
PÂTÉ DE CHEVREUIL   venison pâté
PÂTÉ DE FOIE   liver pâté
PÂTÉ DE FOIE DE PORC   finely ground pork livers
PÂTÉ DE FOIE DE VOLAILLE   chicken liver pâté
PÂTÉ DE FOIE GRAS   goose liver
PÂTÉ DE GIBIER   pâté made with game
PÂTÉ DE GRIVE   pâté made with thrush or songbird
PÂTÉ DE LAPIN   rabbit pâté

PÂTÉ DE LIÈVRE   pâté of wild hare
PÂTÉ DE POISSON   fish pâté
PÂTÉ DE TÊTE   made from calf's head
PÂTÉ EN CROÛTE   mixture covered with pastry
PÂTÉ EN CROÛTE AUX ÉPINARDS   veal, ham and pork
   pie with spinach
PÂTE FEUILLETÉE   puff pastry
PÂTÉ MAISON   house specialty
PÂTES ALIMENTAIRES   spaghetti, macaroni
PÂTISSERIE   pastry
PÂTISSON   orange flavored pastry
PATRON   proprietor
PAUCHOUSE   fresh water fish stew
PAUPIETTE   slice of chicken, fish or meat filled with
   another mixture, rolled up and sautéed
PAUPIETTE DE VEAU   slice of veal, usually filled with a
   mixture and rolled
PAVÉ AU CHOCOLAT   spongecake with chocolate butter
   cream and chocolate icing
PAVOT   poppy seed
PAYSAN   garnish of carrots, turnips, onions, celery and
   bacon
PAYSANNE, À LA   any dish prepared in the country style
PÊCHE   peach
PÊCHE ALEXANDRA   poached peach with ice cream and
   pureed berries
PÊCHE CARDINAL   poached peaches with raspberry puree
PÊCHE MELBA   vanilla ice cream with peaches in
   raspberry puree
PERCE-PIERRE   edible algae growing on rock
PERCHE   lake fish
PERDRIX   partridge
PERDRIX À LA CATALANE   partridge stew
PERDRIX À LA VIGNERONNE   partridges with grapes
PERDRIX AUX CHOUX   casseroled partridge with cabbage
PÉRIGUEUX, SAUCE   brown sauce with tomatoes,
   Madeira and truffles

PÉRIGOURDINE, SAUCE À LA   sauce of truffles and liver

PERLANT   slightly sparkling

PERNOD   before dinner drink which tastes like Absinthe

PERRIER   brand of mineral water

PERSANE, À LA   fried eggplant, onion, peppers and tomato

PERSIL   parsley

PERSILLADE   chopped parsley and garlic

PERSILLE DES ARAVIS   blue-veined, sharp goat's milk cheese

PÉTILLANT   slightly sparkling

PETIT   small

PETIT DÉJEUNER   breakfast

PETIT DÉJEUNER COMPLET   coffee or tea, croissants, bread, butter and jam

PETIT DÉJEUNER SIMPLE   coffee, hot milk and bread

PETIT FOUR   little filled cakes with sugar frosting topped with candied flowers, nuts or chocolate

PETIT GÂTEAU SEC   cookie

PETIT GRATIN DE CRABE AU VIN BLANC   crab meat in white wine sauce baked with cheese

PETIT MILLE-FEUILLE   Napoleon; pastry filled with an almond cream sauce and glazed with a sugary mixture

PETIT PAIN   roll

PETIT PÂTÉ   small pastry filled with ground meat

PETIT PÂTÉ CHAUD   small hot patty filled with meat or fish or grated cheese

PETIT POT   small container or dish

PETIT POT DE CRÈME   little pot of cream, cold custard

PETIT POT DE CRÈME À LA VANILLE   small vanilla custard

PETIT POT DE CRÈME AU CHOCOLAT   chocolate cream custard

PETIT POUSSIN   a very small chicken

PETIT SALÉ   salt pork

PETIT SALÉ AUX LENTILLES   boiled bacon with lentils in a casserole

PETIT SUISSE   miniature cheese, resembling cream cheese

PETITE CAISSE DE FROMAGE   cheese and artichoke appetizers

PETITE MARMITE   clear, strong bouillon with meat, vegetables, grated cheese, served in earthenware pots

PETITES BOUCHÉES   small pastry shells filled with fish or other ingredients

PETITS OIGNONS AUX RAISINS   button onions with raisins

PETITS POIS   peas

PETITS POIS À LA FRANÇAISE   young peas and baby onions

PETITS POIS AU LARD   peas with bacon

PETITS POIS FRAIS   fresh peas braised with onions and butter

PÉTONCLE   tiny scallop

PÉTONCLE, RAGOÛT DE   scallop stew

PETS DE NONNE   small fried pastries

PIBALLES   small eels

PICHET   pitcher or wine decanter

PICODON DE VALRÉAS   goat's milk cheese with a nutty taste

PICON   bitter, orange flavored drink

PIÈCE DE RÉSISTANCE   very special main dish

PIED   foot

PIED DE COCHON   pig's foot

PIED DE MOUTON   stuffed sheep's foot

PIED DE PORC   pig's foot

PIED DE PORC SAINTE-MENEHOULD   grilled pig feet

PIED DE VEAU   calves' feet

PIERRE-QUI-VIRE   tangy cheese with strong smell

PIEUVRE   octopus

PIGEON À LA RUSSE   squab or pigeon cooked with a sour cream sauce

PIGEONNEAU   squab

PIGEONNEAU AUX POIS   baked squab with peas, onions, pork, chicken broth

PIGEONNEAU SUR CANAPÉ   roast squab on liver canape
PIGNON   pine nut
PILAF   rice cooked with onions and broth
PILAW   rice prepared with various other ingredients
PILCHARD   sardine
PIMENT DOUX   sweet red pimento
PIMENT VERT   green pimento
PINEAU DES CHARENTES   sweet wine
PINTADE   guinea fowl
PINTADE AUX LENTILLES   guinea hen with lentils
PINTADE FORESTIÈRE   guinea hen with pork, onions,
   potatoes, broth, mushrooms
PINTADEAU   young guinea fowl
PINTADEAU AUX GIROLLES   stuffed with mushrooms,
   braised in wine
PINTADEAU EN COCOTTE   braised in a casserole
PINTADEAU MONSOLET   stuffed with goose liver,
   braised with artichokes
PINTADEAU RICHELIEU   fried in butter with lemon
   juice
PINTADEAU SALMI   braised with onions, mushrooms,
   Madeira wine
PINTADEAU SOUVAROFF   stuffed with goose liver,
   braised in Madeira wine
PIPERADE   scrambled eggs, pepper, onions, tomatoes and
   ham
PIPPERMINT GET   bright green alcoholic mint drink
PIQUANTE   sharp, spicy
PIQUANTE, SAUCE   spicy, brown sauce with small
   onions and pickles
PIROGUIS   unsweetened pastry filled with meat or
   cheese, usually served hot with soup
PISSALADIÈRE   Provençale onion and anchovy pie
PISTACHE   pistachio nut
PISTOU, SOUPE AU   garlic and vegetable soup with thin
   pasta

PITHIVIERS   puff pastry filled with almond cream and rum

PLAT   serving plate

PLAT DE CÔTES   boiled beef short ribs and vegetables

PLAT DE CÔTES DE PORC RÔTIES   roast spare ribs

PLAT DU JOUR   speciality of the day

PLAT PRINCIPAL   main dish

PLATEAU   tray

PLATEAU DE FROMAGES   cheese platter

PLATEAU DE FRUITS DE MER   seafood platter with raw and cooked shellfish, including oysters, clams, mussels, crabs

PLEUROTE   wild mushroom

PLIE   fish like sole or flounder

PLOMBIÈRES   dessert of vanilla ice cream, candied fruit, kirsch, and sweetened whipped cream

PLOUSE   codfish

POCHÉ   poached

POCHOUSE   freshwater fish stew prepared with white wine

POCHOUSE BOURGUIGNONNE   with eel and other fish in wine

PÔELÉ   fried

POGNE   brioche cake filled with fruit or jam

POGNON   griddle cake

POINT, À   medium rare steak or ripe

POINTES D'ASPERGES   asparagus tips

POIRE   pear

POIRE ALMA   pear poached in wine

POIRE AU GRATIN   pear baked with wine and macaroons

POIRE BELLE HÉLÈNE   pear with vanilla ice cream and chocolate sauce

POIRE CARDINAL   cooked pears with raspberry sauce and toasted almonds

POIRE CONDÉ   hot pear on vanilla flavored rice

POIRE POCHÉE AU VIN ROUGE   pear poached in red wine

POIRE WILLIAMS   pear brandy

POIREAU   leek

POIREAU À LA NIÇOISE   leek stewed with oil and tomatoes

POIS   pea

POIS À LA FRANÇAISE   green peas cooked with onions and lettuce

POIS CASSÉS   split peas

POIS CHICHE   chick-pea

POIS FRAIS, BRAISAGE DE   fresh peas, braised lettuce and scallions

POISON   poison

POISSON   fish

POISSON À LA PROVENÇALE   white fish fried with onions, garlic, tomatoes, fresh herbs

POISSON BASQUE   fish sautéed in clam juice, white wine, mashed tomatoes, scallions

POISSON COCOTTE   swordfish or tuna simmered in a skillet with onions, butter and white wine

POISSON CÔTE D'AZUR   fish simmered with tomatoes, fennel, thyme, garlic, peppercorns and wine

POISSON D'EAU DOUCE   freshwater fish

POISSON DE LAC   lake fish

POISSON DE MER   saltwater fish

POISSON DE RIVIÈRE   river fish

POISSON DU HAVRE, FILETS DE   fish sautéed then flamed with whiskey, clam juice, heavy cream, lemon juice

POISSON FARCI À LA FLORENTINE   baked fish with spinach stuffing

POISSON MAÎTRE D'HÔTEL   fish boiled in saucepan with thin slices of lemon

POISSON MEUNIÈRE   fish sautéed with flour, butter, lemon juice

POISSON ORLY   fish fillets deep fried in batter with tomato sauce

POISSON POCHÉ AU COURT BOUILLON   fish poached in fish stock

POITRINE   breast of meat or poultry

POITRINE D'OIE FUMÉE   smoked goose breast

POITRINE DE MOUTON   breast of mutton

POITRINE DE MOUTON FARCIE   mutton breast stuffed with ham

POITRINE DE VEAU   breast of veal

POITRINE FUMÉE   smoked bacon

POIVRADE, SAUCE   brown sauce dominated with black pepper

POIVRE   pepper

POIVRE BLANC   white pepper

POIVRE D'ÂNE   cheese made with herbs

POIVRE DE CAYENNE   red pepper

POIVRE, GRAINS DE   peppercorns

POIVRE NOIR   black pepper

POIVRON   green or red pepper

POIVRON FARCIS AU RIZ   pepper stuffed with rice

POLENTA   cooked cornmeal, water, butter and cheese

POMME   apple

POMME BELLE VUE   molded apple custard

POMME BONNE FEMME   baked apple

POMME EN L'AIR   caramelized apple slices

POMME SAUVAGE   wild crabapple

POMME DE TERRE   potato

POMMES DE TERRE À L'AIL   potatoes pureed with garlic

POMMES DE TERRE À L'AIL PURÉE DE   garlic mashed potatoes

POMMES DE TERRE À L'ANGLAISE   boiled potatoes

POMMES DE TERRE À L'HUILE   French potato salad, with vinegar, olive oil, herbs

POMMES DE TERRE À LA BOULANGÈRE   potatoes cooked with meat

POMMES DE TERRE À LA LYONNAISE   sautéed potatoes with onions

POMMES DE TERRE À LA SARLADAISE   casserole of potatoes cooked in goose fat

POMMES DE TERRE ALLUMETTES   shoestring potatoes

POMMES DE TERRE ANNA   sliced potatoes baked in butter

POMMES DE TERRE AU GRATIN DAUPHINOIS   baked scalloped potatoes

POMMES DE TERRE BASQUAISE   baked potatoes, stuffed with ham, tomatoes and garlic

POMMES DE TERRE BIGOUDENN   baked slices of unpeeled potato

POMMES DE TERRE BOUILLIES   boiled potatoes

POMMES DE TERRE BRETONNE   potatoes with cream, celery and onions

POMMES DE TERRE BYRON   baked potato pancake

POMMES DE TERRE CHATOUILLARD   deep-fried ribbon potatoes

POMMES DE TERRE CHIPS   potato chips

POMMES DE TERRE, COLLERETTES DE   thin slices of potato, fried

POMMES DE TERRE, CROQUETTES DE   mashed potatoes, deep-fried in breadcrumbs

POMMES DE TERRE DAUPHINE   fried balls of mashed potatoes mixed with pastry

POMMES DE TERRE DAUPHINOISE   baked sliced potatoes, milk, garlic and cheese

POMMES DE TERRE DUCHESSE   mashed potatoes with butter, egg yolks and nutmeg

POMMES DE TERRE EN PAILLE   fried julienned potatoes

POMMES DE TERRE EN ROBE DES CHAMPS   potatoes cooked with skins on

POMMES DE TERRE FRITES   french fried potatoes

POMMES DE TERRE GRATINÉES   potatoes browned with cheese

POMMES DE TERRE LORETTE   fried potato croquettes

POMMES DE TERRE MACAIRE   baked mashed potatoes fried in flat cakes

POMMES DE TERRE MAÎTRE D'HÔTEL   boiled potatoes, then sautéed with hot milk

POMMES DE TERRE MONT-DORÉ   mashed potatoes and cheese baked in the oven

POMMES DE TERRE, MOUSSELINE DE   potatoes pureed with butter, egg yolks and cream

POMMES DE TERRE NATURE   plain boiled potatoes

POMMES DE TERRE PARISIENNE   fried potato balls

POMMES DE TERRE PARMENTIER   large potato cubes sautéed in butter

POMMES DE TERRE PONT-NEUF   classic fries

POMMES DE TERRE, PURÉE DE   mashed potatoes

POMMES DE TERRE RISSOLÉES   sautéed potatoes

POMMES DE TERRE SAVOYARDE AU GRATIN   sliced potatoes baked with cheese

POMMES DE TERRE SOUFFLÉES   slices of potato fried twice to fluff up

POMMES DE TERRE ST. FLOUR   sliced potatoes with bacon baked on cabbage leaves

POMMES DE TERRE VAPEUR   steamed or boiled potatoes

POMMES DE TERRE VOISIN   potato cake of sliced potato and cheese

POMMES DE TERRE YVETTE   baked potato strips

POMPETTES   orange flavored sweet pastry

POMPONNETTE   ground meat or poultry in a pastry case

PONT-L'ÉVÊQUE   strong soft cheese

PORC   pork

PORC, CARRÉ DE   rib roast of pork

PORC, CÔTE DE   loin chop of pork

PORC, ÉCHINE DE   pork spare rib

PORC MARENGO   pork stewed with wine and tomatoes

PORC, PLAT DE CÔTE DE spare ribs
PORCELET young suckling pig
PORT SALUT fairly mild, semi-hard cheese
PORTO port
PORTUGAISE thick soup with pimentos and tomatoes
PORTUGAISES elongated, crinkle shell oysters
POT-AU-FEU broth in which meat and vegetables are
  cooked
POT-AU-FEU À LA NORMANDE boiled dinner of beef,
  pork, veal or chicken, with vegetables
POT-AU-FEU D'HOMARD lobster and seafood stew
POT-DE-CRÈME individual custard dessert
POTAGE soup, also see potée, consommé
POTAGE À LA REINE cream of chicken
POTAGE AU VERMICELLE noodle soup
POTAGE AUX LENTILLES lentil soup
POTAGE DE VOLAILLE chicken broth
POTAGE DU JOUR soup of the day
POTAGE HONGROIS goulash soup
POTAGE OXTAIL oxtail soup
POTAGE PORTUGAIS tomato soup
POTAGE ST. CLOUD thick soup of pureed peas with
  croutons
POTAGE ST. GERMAIN pea soup
POTÉE thick stew-like soup
POTÉE BOURGUIGNONNE thick stew of vegetables,
  pork and sausage
POTÉE CHAMPENOISE stew of ham, bacon, sausage
  and cabbage
POTÉE COMTOISE soup of cabbage, potato and sausage
POTÉE LIMOUSINE stew made of pork, chestnuts and
  red cabbage
POTÉE LORRAINE stew of pork, sausage, cabbage
POTIRON pumpkin
POUDING pudding
POULARDE large roasting chicken

POULARDE À L'ÉCREVISSES   chicken with crayfish in wine and cream sauce

POULARDE AU RIESLING   coq au vin, made with white wine instead of red

POULARDE AU VINAIGRE   chicken, tomatoes, wine, vinegar and cream sauce

POULARDE BASQUAISE   chicken with peppers, mushrooms, eggplant

POULARDE BAYONNAISE   roasting hen with onions

POULARDE CÉLESTINE   chicken with mushrooms in a wine and cream sauce

POULARDE CHEVALIÈRE   chicken in pastry with mushrooms

POULARDE DE BRESSE EN BRIOCHE   chicken baked in a yeast dough

POULARDE DEMI DEUIL   with truffles, simmered in broth with cream sauce

POULARDE DEMI-DÉSOSSÉE   half-boned chicken

POULARDE DERBY   chicken with rice, foie gras, truffles, wine

POULARDE EN CHEMISE   poached stuffed chicken

POULARDE LYONNAISE   stuffed chicken with truffles, vegetables

POULARDE MÈRE FILLIOUX   with sausage and sweetbreads, cooked in a cream sauce

POULARDE PAYSANNE   chicken in sauce with vegetables, bacon and potatoes

POULARDE STRASBOURGEOISE   chicken breasts stuffed with ground goose livers

POULE   hen, also see poulet and poularde

POULE AU POT   chicken in the pot, chicken soup

POULE AU POT HENRI IV   stuffed chicken cooked in wine

POULE FAISANE   female pheasant

POULE IVOIRE   boiled fowl with cream sauce

POULET   chicken, also see poularde and poule

POULET À L'ARMAGNAC   chicken with white cream
sauce and Armagnac brandy

POULET À LA CASSEROLE   chicken sautéed in a skillet

POULET À LA CRÈME   chicken in cream sauce

POULET À LA NIÇOISE   chicken cooked with garlic,
saffron and tomatoes

POULET À LA PARISIENNE   sautéed chicken with
mashed potatoes in wine

POULET À LA ROUILLEUSE   chicken in wine and garlic
sauce

POULET ALEXANDRA   sautéed chicken with cream
sauce

POULET AU VIN JAUNE   chicken in a cream sauce made
with wine

POULET BARBOUILLÉ   chicken in wine sauce

POULET BASQUAISE   chicken with tomatoes and sweet
peppers

POULET BEAULIEU   chicken in artichokes, potatoes and
wine sauce

POULET BOIVIN   sautéed chicken with artichokes

POULET BORDEAUX   fried with tomatoes, wine and
mushrooms

POULET CHASSEUR   sautéed with shallots and tomato
sauce

POULET COCOTTE   baked chicken with pork, onions,
potatoes, artichoke hearts, chicken broth

POULET COCOTTE BONNE FEMME   baked chicken
with potatoes and bacon

POULET COMPOTE   chicken stew

POULET DIJON   sautéed with wine, Dijon style mustard,
sour cream

POULET DUC   chicken sautéed with brandy in heavy
cream and wine

POULET EN GELÉE   jellied tarragon chicken

POULET FARCI   stuffed with ham, liver and cooked in
soup

POULET FORESTIÈRE   sautéed with mushrooms, potatoes and Madeira

POULET FRIT   fried chicken

POULET GRILLÉ À LA DIABLE   broiled with mustard, herb and breadcrumbs

POULET GRILLÉ NATUREL   plain broiled chicken

POULET KATOFF   grilled chicken served on mashed potatoes

POULET KIEV   deep fried breast of chicken stuffed with seasoned butter

POULET MARENGO   chicken sautéed in olive oil, with mushrooms, tomatoes

POULET MATELOTE   chicken in red wine

POULET NEVA   chicken stuffed with ground chicken liver in aspic

POULET POCHÉ AU RIZ   boiled chicken with rice

POULET POCHÉ AUX AROMATES   chicken simmered in white wine and vegetables

POULET RÔTI   roast chicken

POULET RÔTI À L'ÉSTRAGON   chicken with tarragon cream sauce

POULET RÔTI AU BEURRE   chicken roasted in butter

POULET SAUTÉ À LA BORDELAISE   sautéed chicken with artichoke hearts

POULET SAUTÉ ARLÉSIEN   fried chicken with eggplant in white wine

POULET SAUTÉ AU VIN BLANC   chicken in cream and white wine

POULET SAUTÉ PARMENTIER   chicken sautéed with potatoes in wine

POULET VALLÉE D'AUGE   chicken with apples

POULETTE, SAUCE   creamy white sauce made with egg yolks

POULPE   octopus

POURBOIRE   tip

POUSSEZ   push

POUSSIN   baby chicken, also see poule, poulet, poularde

POUTARGUE   paste of mullet roe
POUTINA NONNAT   very small fried fish
PRAIRE   small clam
PRALIN   brittle of almonds, walnuts hazelnuts, pecans
   and caramel
PRALIN DE NOIX   caramelized walnut brittle
PRÉ-SALÉ   distinctive tasting salt marsh lamb
PRESSION, BIÈRE   draft beer
PRINTANIÈRE   with vegetable garnish
PRINTANIÈRE, SAUCE   white sauce with green vegetables
PRIVÉ   private
PRIX FIXE   fixed price
PROFITEROLES   pastry filled with ice cream and topped
   with chocolate sauce
PROPRIÉTÉ PRIVÉE   private property
PROVENÇALE, À LA   with garlic, tomatoes and olive oil
PRUNE   plum
PRUNEAUX   dried prunes
PUITS D'AMOUR   pastry shell with liqueur flavored
   custard
PURÉE BRETONNE   pureed bean soup
PURÉE DE LÉGUME   finely creamed vegetable
PURÉE DE POIS CASSÉS   split pea soup
PURÉE DE POMMES   applesauce
PURÉE SOUBISE   creamed onions
PURÉE ST. GERMAIN   creamed green peas

Q

QUENELLE   dumpling, usually of veal, fish or poultry
QUENELLE DE BROCHET   dumpling of ground pike
QUENELLE DE POISSON   puree of fish formed into balls
   and poached
QUETSCH   small purple plum
QUETSCH   liquor distilled from plums
QUEUE   tail
QUEUE DE BOEUF   oxtail

QUEUE DE BOEUF FARCIE   stuffed oxtail
QUEUE DE BOEUF, POTAGE DE   oxtail soup
QUEUES D'ÉCRIVISSES   crayfish tails
QUICHE   tart with egg and cream, meat or vegetable
   filling
QUICHE AU FROMAGE   cheese quiche
QUICHE DE CREVETTES   shrimp quiche
QUICHE LORRAINE   egg and cheese pie
QUIMPER   mackerel

R

RÂBLE DE LIÈVRE   saddle of rabbit
RABOTE   apple in pastry
RACLETTE   melted cheese with boiled potatoes, pickles
   and pickled onions
RADIS   radish
RAFRAÎCHIS, FRUITS   chilled fruit salad
RAGOÛT   stew, usually of meat
RAGOÛT BIGOUDEN   stewed sausage with potato and
   onions
RAIE   skate-like fish
RAIE AU BEURRE NOIR   skate with black butter
RAIFORT   horseradish
RAISIN   grape
RAISIN DE CORINTHE   raisin
RAISINÉ   grape jelly
RAÏTO   fish sauce of red wine, tomatoes, garlic and capers
RAMEQUIN   melted cheese, like a fondue
RAMEQUIN AU FROMAGE   cheese tarts
RAMEQUIN FORESTIÈRE   thick sauce of eggs, cheese
   and mushrooms baked until brown
RANCIO   dessert wine
RÂPÉ, FROMAGE   grated cheese
RÂPÉE À LA MORVANDELLE   grated potato baked with
   eggs and cheese
RASCASSE   Mediterranean fish used for soup and stews

RATATOUILLE   stewed squash, tomatoes, vegetables and garlic

RATATOUILLE NIÇOISE   eggplant, onions, tomatoes and peppers stewed in oil

RAVIGOTTE, SAUCE   cream sauce with shallots, herbs and spices

RAVIOLES   pastries from goats' cheese

REBLOCHON   semi-hard cheese

RÉGLISSE   liquorice

REGUIGNEU   fried country ham

REINE CLAUDE   plum

REINE DE SABA   chocolate, rum and almond cake

REINE, À LA   with mince meat or fowl

RELAIS ROUTIER   roadside restaurant

RENSEIGNEMENTS   information

REPAS   meal

RÉSERVÉ   reserved

RHUBARBE   rhubarb

RHUM   rum

RICARD   aperitif of wine with aniseed, like Pernod

RICHELIEU   almond pastry with apricot jam and almond cream

RIGOTTE CONDRIEU   soft and mild cheese with a milky taste

RILLETTE   soft, spreadable pork or goose paste

RILLETTE DE LAPIN   made of pork and rabbit

RILLETTE DE TOURS   ground up pork meat, somewhat coarser than pâté

RILLETTES DE PORC   soft potted pork

RIS D'AGNEAU   lamb sweetbreads

RIS D'AGNEAU BRAISÉ   braised lamb sweetbreads

RIS DE VEAU   veal sweetbreads

RIS DE VEAU À LA CRÈME   braised sweetbreads in cream

RIS DE VEAU À LA SUÉDOISE   sweetbreads, tongue and horseradish sauce

RIS DE VEAU AU BEURRE NOIR   sweetbreads in brown butter sauce

RIS DE VEAU GUIZOT   braised sweetbreads

RISOTTO   rice braised in chicken stock with tomatoes and parmesan cheese

RISOTTO À LA PIÉMONTAISE   rice braised in chicken stock

RISSOLE   ground mixture covered with pastry and deep fried

RIZ   rice

RIZ À L'ÉTUVÉE AU BEURRE   steamed and buttered rice

RIZ À LA CRÉOLE   boiled rice with tomatoes and pimentos

RIZ AU LAIT   rice custard

RIZ COMPLET   brown rice

RIZ IMPÉRATRICE   Bavarian cream with rice, fruits and Kirsch

RIZ PILAF   rice boiled in a bouillon

RIZ SAUVAGE   wild rice

RIZ VALENCIENNE   rice, tomatoes, saffron, onions and shellfish

ROBERT, SAUCE   brown sauce made with onions, wine and vinegar

ROCHES   large Portuguese oyster

ROGNON   kidney

ROGNON BLANC   testicle

ROGNON DE MOUTON   sheep kidney

ROGNON DE VEAU   veal kidney

ROGNON DE VEAU À LA LIÉGOISE   calf's kidneys, juniper berries and gin

ROGNON DE VEAU EN CASSEROLE   kidney in butter and mustard sauce

ROGNON DE VEAU FLAMBÉ   sautéed kidney flambéed with mushroom sauce

ROGNON EN BROCHETTE   lambs' kidneys on a skewer

ROGNON EN CASSEROLE   sautéed kidneys with mustard sauce

ROGNON SAUTÉ FLAMBÉ   veal and lamb kidney, sautéed and flambéed

ROGNON SAUTÉ MADÈRE   sautéed kidney with wine
ROGNONNADE   veal loin with kidneys attached
ROLLMOPS   pickled herring around a piece of onion
ROLLOT   soft, cow's milk cheese, tangy taste
ROMAINE   romaine lettuce
ROMARIN   rosemary
ROMSTECK   rump steak
ROQUEFORT   blue-veined, moist, salty, tangy cheese of
   ewe's milk
ROSBIF   roast beef
ROSETTE   large pork sausage served in slices
ROSETTE DE BOEUF   dried sausage
RÔTI   roast
RÔTI DE BOEUF JARDINIÈRE   roast beef with vegetables
RÔTI DE BOEUF PÔELÉ MATIGNON   roast beef with
   vegetables and potatoes
RÔTI, FILET   roasted fillet
RÔTI, FOIE   roasted liver
RÔTI, JARRET   roasted knuckle
RÔTI, ROGNON   roasted kidneys
RÔTIE   slice of toast
RÔTISSERIE   restaurant specializing in grilled meat
ROUELLE DE VEAU   veal shank
ROUENNAISE, SAUCE   brown sauce containing ground
   duck livers
ROUGET   red Mediterranean fish
ROUGET AU FENOUIL   rouget cooked with olive oil,
   bacon and fennel
ROUGET MEUNIÈRE   red mullet fried in butter
ROUILLE   spicy sauce with olive oil, red peppers,
   tomatoes and garlic served with fish soups
ROUILLE (SAUCE)   thick, spicy sauce with olive oil, hot
   peppers, tomatoes, garlic, served with fish soups
ROULÉ   rolled
ROUSSETTE   sweet corn flour fritter made with brandy
ROUX   butter and flour used as a thickener
ROYAN   pilchard, similar to herring or sardine

RUMSTECK   rumpsteak
RUSSE   with sour cream

S

SABAYON   sweet sauce of egg yolks, sugar, wine and
   flavoring
SABLÉ   shortbread cookie
SABODET   sausage from pig's head
SAFRAN   saffron
SAIGNANT   rare steak
SAINT-PIERRE   sea fish
SAISON, DE   in season
SALADE   salad
SALADE À LA BOUCHÈRE   boiled beef, potatoes,
   tomatoes
SALADE ALBIGNAC   crayfish or chicken salad
SALADE ALLEMANDE   salad of apple, herring and
   potato
SALADE ARLÉSIENNE   potatoes, artichokes, anchovies
   and tomatoes
SALADE CAUCHOISE   potato, celery and ham salad
SALADE CHIFFONNADE   shredded lettuce and sorrel in
   melted butter
SALADE COMPOSÉE   main course combination salad
SALADE D'ENDIVES   endive salad
SALADE D'ENDIVES ET DE BETTERAVES   endive and
   beet salad
SALADE DE BOEUF À LA PARISIENNE   beef and potato
   salad
SALADE DE CÉLERI   celery root in mustard mayonnaise
   dressing
SALADE DE CERVELAS   white sausage in vinaigrette
   sauce
SALADE DE COEURS D'ARTICHAUTS   artichoke hearts
   in oil and vinegar
SALADE DE CONCOMBRES   cucumber salad

SALADE DE FRUITS   fruit salad
SALADE DE HARENG   herring salad
SALADE DE LAITUE   lettuce
SALADE DE MOULES   mussel salad
SALADE DE MOULES À LA PROVENÇALE   mussel salad with chopped onion fried in olive oil with tomatoes and garlic
SALADE DE MUSEAU DE BOEUF   marinated beef headcheese
SALADE DE NOIX   nut and cheese salad
SALADE DE PISSENLITS AU LARD   dandelion leaves, bacon and new potatoes
SALADE DE POMMES DE TERRE   boiled potatoes, oil and vinegar dressing
SALADE DE QUEUES D'ÉCREVISSES   crayfish salad
SALADE DE RIZ À L'ORIENTALE   oriental rice salad
SALADE DE THON   tuna salad
SALADE DE TOMATES   tomato salad
SALADE DE VOLAILLE   chicken salad with mayonnaise
SALADE FLAMANDE   potato salad with salt herring
SALADE FOLLE   mixed salad, usually including green beans and liver
SALADE FRANCILLON   salad of mussels and marinated potato
SALADE ITALIENNE   potatoes, asparagus tips, mayonnaise with anchovies, salami, olives, capers
SALADE JAPONAISE   tomato, orange and pineapple with sour cream
SALADE LYONNAISE   cooked diced vegetables, anchovies, oil and vinegar, onions, capers and hard eggs
SALADE MADRAS   rice salad with tomatoes, green peppers, mustard, salad oil, wine vinegar, cooked rice
SALADE MÊLÉE   mixed salad
SALADE MIMOSA   green salad with vinaigrette, sieved egg and herbs
SALADE NIÇOISE   salad with olives, anchovies, tuna fish
SALADE PANACHÉE   mixed salad

SALADE PAYSAN   quartered tomatoes, chopped onion, cucumbers, anchovies, oil and vinegar

SALADE PERNOLLET   truffle and crayfish salad

SALADE PORT ROYAL   apples, beans, potatoes, mayonnaise, hard-boiled eggs

SALADE POTAGER   garden vegetable salad

SALADE RAPHAËL   lettuce, cucumber, asparagus, tomatoes, radishes and sauce

SALADE RUSSE   cooked vegetables in mayonnaise

SALADE SHEPHERDESS   rice salad with hard-boiled eggs, scallions, horseradish, sour cream

SALADE TOURANGELLE   green bean and potato salad

SALADE VARIÉE   mixed salad

SALADE VERTE   green salad

SALADE VIGNERON   lettuce hearts with sour cream

SALADE WALDORF   apples, celery and walnuts in mayonnaise

SALADIER   salad bowl

SALAMBO   small cake filled with kirsch-cream

SALDA   soup of bacon, sausage, cabbage and beans

SALÉ   salted

SALMIS   stewlike preparation of game birds or poultry in wine

SALMIS DE PALOMBES   roast pigeon, wine, onions, ham and mushrooms

SALMIS DE POISSONS   mixed seafood stew with wine

SALPICON   diced vegetables, meat and/or fish in a sauce

SALPICON DE VOLAILLE   diced turkey or chicken in white wine sauce

SANCIAU   thick pancake

SANDRE   perchlike freshwater fish

SANDWICH MIXTE   gruyère cheese and ham on a baguette

SANGLIER   wild boar

SANGLIER, CUISSOT DE   haunch

SANGLIER, SELLE DE   saddle

SANTE   leek, potato and vegetable soup

SANTÉ! (À VOTRE)   cheers

SARCELLE   teal, small duck

SARDINE   small fish

SARDINE À L'HUILE   sardine in olive oil

SARDINE NIÇOISE   boneless sardine cooked in white wine, mushrooms and spices

SARDINES AUX OEUFS AU CITRON   sardines with hard boiled eggs and lemon

SAUCE   liquid dressing for food

SAUCE À LA CRESSONADE   watercress sauce

SAUCE À LA DIABLE   spicy sauce with white wine

SAUCE AIGRELETTE   tart sauce

SAUCE AÏLLADA   oil and garlic sauce

SAUCE ALBERT   creamed horseradish sauce

SAUCE ALBERTINE   sauce made with mushrooms and white wine

SAUCE ALLEMANDE   cream sauce with egg yolks and lemon juice

SAUCE AMIRAL   anchovy and herb sauce

SAUCE ANCIENNE   cream sauce with mushrooms and wine

SAUCE ARMENONVILLE   sauce of potatoes, tomatoes and artichokes

SAUCE AURORE   creamy sauce with tomato puree

SAUCE AUX CÂPRES   sauce made from fish concentrate, capers and butter

SAUCE AUX FRAISES   fresh strawberry sauce

SAUCE AUX FRAMBOISES   fresh raspberry sauce

SAUCE AUX RIS DE VEAU À LA SUÉDOISE   sweetbreads, tongue and horseradish sauce

SAUCE BÉARNAISE   sauce of egg yolks, butter, shallots, tarragon, white wine, vinegar, herbs

SAUCE BÉCHAMEL   creamy white sauce with buttermilk

SAUCE BERCY   shallots, white wine in a creamy chicken sauce

SAUCE BIGARADE   orange sauce

SAUCE BOLOGNAISE   sauce of tomatoes and vegetables, heavy garlic

SAUCE BONNE FEMME   shallots, white wine, mushrooms and lemon juice

SAUCE BORDELAISE   brown sauce of shallots, red wine and bone marrow

SAUCE BRETONNE   creamy white sauce with strips of vegetables

SAUCE BRUNE   brown sauce from meat stock, onions and tomatoes

SAUCE CAFÉ DE PARIS   cream, mustard and herbs

SAUCE CARDINAL   sauce of cream with lobster pieces and herbs

SAUCE CHADEAU   sweet dessert sauce

SAUCE CHASSEUR   brown sauce with wine, mushrooms, onions

SAUCE CHIVRY   white wine sauce with herbs

SAUCE CHORON   tomato flavored béarnaise sauce

SAUCE COLLIOURE   anchovy and mayonnaise sauce

SAUCE CRAPAUDINE   brown sauce made with onions, vinegar and spices

SAUCE DEMI GLACÉ   concentrated sauce lightened with consommé

SAUCE DIANE   peppery cream sauce

SAUCE DUGLÈRE   white sauce with shallots, white wine, tomatoes

SAUCE EN MEURETTE   red wine sauce

SAUCE ESPAGNOLE   vegetable, meat and tomato sauce

SAUCE FINANCIÈRE   cream, wine, spices, mushrooms, olives, truffles

SAUCE FORESTIÈRE   mushroom sauce

SAUCE GAILLARDE   hard egg yolks, oil, vinegar, capers, pickles

SAUCE GASTRONOME   dark sauce made with white wine

SAUCE GENEVOISE   sauce of fish stock, red wine and anchovy

SAUCE GENOISE   cold sauce of nuts, cream and mayonnaise

SAUCE GRAND VENEUR   pepper sauce with red currant jelly and cream

SAUCE GRIBICHE   hard-boiled egg yolks with oil, vinegar, pickles

SAUCE HOLLANDAISE   sauce of egg yolks, butter and lemon juice

SAUCE HONGROISE   white sauce with onions and paprika

SAUCE INDIENNE   with rice or curry

SAUCE ITALIENNE   brown sauce with mushrooms, ham and tarragon

SAUCE JOURNEAUX   chicken liver sauce

SAUCE LIVORNAISE   olive oil, egg yolks and anchovy paste

SAUCE MADÈRE   meat stock with Madeira wine

SAUCE MALTAISE   hollandaise sauce with grated orange peel

SAUCE MARCHAND DE VIN   dark brown sauce made with meat and wine

SAUCE MARGUERY   white wine and seafood sauce

SAUCE MATELOTE   fish sauce made with wine, anchovies and mushrooms

SAUCE MIRABEAU   anchovies, garlic, lemon juice

SAUCE MORNAY   creamy cheese sauce with eggs

SAUCE MOUSSELINE   hollandaise sauce with whipped cream

SAUCE MOUSSEUSE   butter with lemon juice and whipped cream

SAUCE NANTUA   white wine shrimp sauce with shrimp butter

SAUCE NAPOLITAINE   horseradish, red currant jelly and Madeira

SAUCE NESSELRODE   sauce containing fruits and chestnuts

SAUCE NIÇOISE   tomato and meat sauce

SAUCE NOISETTE   egg yolks and lemon in cream with butter added

SAUCE NORMANDE   fish cream sauce with mushrooms
SAUCE PARISIENNE   cream cheese, oil and lemon juice
SAUCE PAUVRE HOMME   stock, vinegar, shallots and breadcrumbs
SAUCE PÉRIGOURDINE   sauce with truffles and liver
SAUCE PÉRIGUEUX   brown sauce with tomatoes, Madeira wine and truffles
SAUCE PIBRONATA   spicy tomato and pepper sauce
SAUCE PIÉMONTAISE   onions, truffles, pine kernels and garlic
SAUCE PIQUANTE   spicy brown sauce with small onions and pickles
SAUCE POIVRADE   brown sauce dominated with pepper
SAUCE PORTUGAISE   tomato sauce with onions, garlic
SAUCE POULETTE   creamy white sauce with egg yolks
SAUCE PRINTANIÈRE   white sauce with green vegetables
SAUCE RAIFORT   horseradish sauce
SAUCE RAITO   fish sauce of red wine, tomatoes, garlic and walnuts
SAUCE RAVIGOTE   green herb sauce
SAUCE RÉMOULADE   mayonnaise, capers, mustard, anchovies
SAUCE RICHE   white sauce with lobster, butter and truffles
SAUCE ROBERT   sauce of white wine, onion and mustard
SAUCE ROUENNAISE   red wine sauce with liver
SAUCE ROUMAINE   spicy, sweet brown sauce with currants
SAUCE ROYALE   white chicken sauce
SAUCE RUSSE   white sauce with mustard, sugar and lemon juice
SAUCE SABAYON   sweet sauce of egg yolks, sugar, wine
SAUCE SAUPIQUET   spicy wine and vinegar sauce thickened with bread
SAUCE SMITANE   onion and heavy sour cream sauce
SAUCE SOUBISE   onion cream sauce

SAUCE ST. MALO   onions, mushrooms, mustard, anchovy

SAUCE STUFFATU   meat sauce of tomatoes, onions and wine with pasta

SAUCE SUPRÊME   thick chicken stock base

SAUCE TARTARE   mayonnaise, pickles, chives, capers and olives

SAUCE TOULONNAISE   onions, wine, pickle, capers and olives

SAUCE VALENCIENNE   tomato, rice, mushrooms, tongue and cheese

SAUCE VELOUTÉ   cream sauce usually made from chicken and vegetables

SAUCE VERTE   green sauce made from green vegetables with mayonnaise

SAUCE VINCENT   green herb mayonnaise sauce

SAUCISSE   small fresh sausage

SAUCISSE À LA CATALANE   sausage fried with garlic

SAUCISSE CHAUDE   warm sausage

SAUCISSE DE FRANCFORT   hot dog

SAUCISSE DE LYON   boiled coarse grained sausage

SAUCISSE DE STRASBOURG   red skinned hot dog

SAUCISSE DE TOULOUSE   mild country style pork sausage

SAUCISSE GRILLÉE   fried sausage

SAUCISSE PAYSANNE   country style sausage

SAUCISSE, TIMBALE DE   sausage pâté in crust

SAUCISSON   large, dry salami-like sausage

SAUCISSON À L'AIL   garlic sausage served warm

SAUCISSON CERVELAS   garlicky cured pork sausage

SAUCISSON CONFIT   duck, goose, pork cooked and preserved in its own fat

SAUCISSON COU D'OIE FARCI   neck skin of goose, stuffed with meat

SAUCISSON CRÉPINETTE   small sausage patty

SAUCISSON D'ARLES   dried, salami type sausage

SAUCISSON DE CAMPAGNE   country style sausage

SAUCISSON DE LYON   dried pork sausage with garlic, pepper and pork fat

SAUCISSON DE TOULOUSE   pork sausage, boiled then grilled

SAUCISSON EN BRIOCHE   sausage cooked in dough

SAUCISSON EN CROÛTE   sausage cooked in pastry crust

SAUCISSON SEC   dried sausage

SAUCISSONS VARIÉS   slices of mixed sausage

SAUGE   sage

SAUMON   salmon

SAUMON ALSATIEN   salmon boiled in wine and onions over creamed spinach

SAUMON D'ÉCOSSE   Scottish salmon

SAUMON DE NORVÈGE   cold salmon slices in aspic

SAUMON DU RHIN   Rhine salmon

SAUMON FUMÉ   smoked salmon

SAUMON GLACÉ   cold salmon in aspic jelly

SAUMON PATRICIENNE   salmon on toast with glazed sauce

SAUMON POCHÉ   poached whole salmon

SAUMON ROSE À LA PARISIENNE   cold poached salmon on mayonnaise and vegetables

SAUPIQUET   spicy wine and vinegar sauce thickened with bread

SAUTÉ   browned over high heat

SAUTÉ BOEUF   beef cooked in red wine and tomatoes

SAUTÉ DE LAPIN AU VIN BLANC   rabbit stewed in white wine sauce

SAUTÉ DE PORC AUX CHAMPIGNONS   pork sautéed with mushrooms

SAUTÉ DE VEAU   veal browned lightly in fat

SAUTÉ DE VEAU AUX CHAMPIGNONS   veal sautéed with mushrooms

SAUTER   to sauté

SAUTERELLE   shrimp

SAVARIN   ring cake soaked in rum or kirsch

SAVARIN CHANTILLY   cake with Kirsch, jam and whipped cream

SAVOYARDE   vegetable soup with grated cheese

SCAMPI   shellfish similar to shrimp prepared with garlic

SCAROLE   escarole

SCHIFELA   pork with pickled turnips

SCHWEPPES   tonic water

SEAU GLACÉ   ice-bucket

SEC   dry

SEICHE   large squid or cuttlefish

SEIGLE   rye or rye bread

SEL   salt

SELLE D'AGNEAU RÔTIE À LA PERSILLADE   roast saddle of lamb with parsley

SELON GROSSEUR   price according to size, abbreviated s.g.

SERPOLET   wild thyme

SERVICE COMPRIS   tip included, usually 12% to 15%

SERVICE NON COMPRIS   tip not included

SERVIETTE   napkin

SIROP   syrup

SMITANE   sauce of cream, onions, white wine and lemon juice

SOBRONADE   thick soup of pork, white beans, turnips and onions

SOCCA   chick-pea pancake

SOISSONNAISE, SOUPE   haricot bean soup

SOISSONS, HARICOTS DE   dried or fresh white beans

SOLE   flat flounder like fish

SOLE ARLÉSIENNE   sole cooked with garlic, tomatoes and onions

SOLE AU GRATIN   baked sole with shallots, mushrooms and breadcrumbs

SOLE AU VIN BLANC   sole cooked in cream, egg yolks and white wine

SOLE CHAUCHAT   poached sole in Mornay sauce with fried potatoes

SOLE COLBERT   fillets of sole, covered with breadcrumbs and fried

SOLE CUBAT   poached sole with pureed mushrooms in cream sauce

SOLE INDIENNE   tomatoes, coconut milk, cream and curry powder

SOLE MARGUERY   sole, shrimps and mushrooms with a cream sauce

SOLE MÉNAGÈRE   sole baked on vegetables with red wine

SOLE MURAT   sole fried with potatoes and artichoke

SOLE NORMANDE   sole poached in wine in cream sauce with oysters, crayfish

SOLE OLGA   poached sole stuffed into baked potatoes with a covering of shrimp sauce

SOLE SYLVETTE   sole sautéed with vegetables and sherry

SOLFERINO   thick soup of pureed tomatoes, leeks and potatoes

SOMMELIER   wine steward

SON   bran flour

SONNEZ   ring

SORBET   sherbet made with water

SORTIE   exit

SOUBISE   puree of onions and rice

SOUBISE, SAUCE   onion cream sauce

SOUCOUPE   saucer

SOUFFLÉ   light, sweet or piquant mixture served either hot or cold, containing whipped egg whites to puff up when baked

SOUFFLÉ À L'ORANGE, FLAMBÉ   rum, orange and macaroon soufflé, flambéed

SOUFFLÉ AU CHOCOLAT   chocolate soufflé

SOUFFLÉ AU FROMAGE   cheese soufflé in ramekins

SOUFFLÉ AU FROMAGE OEUFS MOLLETS   cheese soufflé with boiled eggs

SOUFFLÉ AU HOMARD   lobster soufflé

SOUFFLÉ AUX FRAMBOISES   raspberry soufflé

SOUFFLÉ AUX FRUITS   soufflé made with fruit preserves or pieces of fruit

SOUFFLÉ DE LÉGUMES   puree of cooked vegetables

SOUFFLÉ GRAND MARNIER   orange liqueur soufflé

SOUFFLÉ MOUSSELINE   cheese soufflé made with cream

SOUFFLÉ NORMAND   soufflé with calvados and apples

SOUFFLÉ OMELETTE   puffy omelet

SOUFFLÉ PALMYRE   soufflé made with macaroons or cake crumbs

SOUFFLÉ REINE   soufflé of poultry or meat

SOUFFLÉ ROTHSCHILD   vanilla soufflé with fruit

SOUPE   peasant style soup, also see consommé, potée and potage

SOUPE À L'AIL   garlic soup

SOUPE À L'OIGNON   onion soup

SOUPE À L'OIGNON GRATINÉE   onion soup gratinéed with cheese

SOUPE À L'OIGNON, MAISON   homemade French onion soup

SOUPE À L'OSEILLE   sorrel soup

SOUPE À LA BIÈRE   beer and onion soup

SOUPE AU PISTOU   vegetable soup with garlic, basil and cheese

SOUPE AUX CERISES   hot cherry soup

SOUPE AUX CHOUX   cabbage soup

SOUPE AUX CUISSES DE GRENOUILLES   frogs' legs soup

SOUPE AUX LÉGUMES   vegetable soup

SOUPE AUX MOULES   cream of mussel soup

SOUPE BERGER   onion and garlic soup

SOUPE DE POISSONS   soup of pureed fish with hot chili and garlic

SOUPE DE POULET   chicken soup

SOUPE DU JOUR   soup of the day

SOUPE ÉPAUTRE   soup stew with meat, vegetables and garlic

SOUPE MONTAGNARDE   thick vegetable soup with cheese

SOUPE ORLÉANAISE   potato soup flavored with green
   herbs
SOUPE PÊCHEUR   fish soup
SOUPE REINE   chicken soup with rice
SOUPE VENDANGES   country soup of meat and
   vegetables
SPAETZLE   small noodle dumplings
SPUMONI   mixed flavored ice cream with candied fruit
ST-FLORENTIN   tangy, soft cheese like cream cheese
ST-GERMAIN   with peas
ST-HONORÉ   iced pastry puffs around cream filled pastry
   ring
ST-MARCELLIN   strong, creamy cheese
ST-MARCELLIN, TOMME DE   soft and mild cheese
ST-MAURE   creamy, strong goat cheese
ST-PAULIN   semi-hard cheese
ST-PIERRE   mild, flat, white ocean fish
ST-RAPHAËL   quinine flavored aperitif
ST-REMY   strong smelling spicy cow's milk cheese
STEAK   steak
STEAK À POINT   steak cooked medium
STEAK AU FOUR   steak baked with herbs
STEAK BIEN CUIT   well-done steak
STEAK DIANE   steak sautéed with wine and peppercorns
STEAK HACHÉ   hamburger steak
STEAK MAÎTRE D'HÔTEL   grilled or pan-fried steak
STEAK POIVRÉ   steak with crushed peppercorns
STEAK SAIGNANT   very rare
STEAK SAUTÉ HENRI IV   fillet steaks with artichokes or
   mushrooms, béarnaise sauce
STEAK TARTARE   raw, chopped onions, capers,
   worcestire sauce and raw egg served on top
STOCAFICADA   dried salt cod stewed in oil with
   vegetables
SUBRIC   croquette of ground meat or fish fried in butter
SUCCÈS AU PRALIN   cake flavored with caramelized
   almonds and frosted with meringue and butter cream

SUCÉE   petit-four containing candied fruit
SUCRE   sugar
SUPÉRIEUR   high alcohol content
SUPRÊME   boneless breast of poultry or a fillet of fish
SUPRÊME DE VOLAILLE   chicken breasts poached in
    butter, wine and cream sauce
SUPRÊME DE VOLAILLE ÉCOSSAISE   chicken breasts
    with vegetables
SUR COMMANDE   special order
SURLONGE   sirloin
SUSPENS   ice cream covered with chopped nuts
SUZE   bitter liqueur

T

TABLE D'HÔTE   proprietor's table or host's table
TACAUD   type of codfish
TAGINE   spicy stew of veal, lamb, chicken and
    vegetables
TALIBUR   apple in pastry
TANCHE   variety of carp
TAPENADE   black olives, anchovies, capers, olive oil,
    lemon juice and tuna fish
TARIF DES CONSOMMATIONS   price list in a bar
TARTE   tart
TARTE À L'ALSACIENNE   custard fruit tart
TARTE À L'OIGNON   onion tart
TARTE À LA TOMATE   custard and tomato pie
TARTE AUX ÉPINARDS   pastry shell filled with creamed
    spinach
TARTE AUX FRAISES   fresh strawberry flan
TARTE AUX FRUITS   fruit tart
TARTE AUX POMMES   apple tart
TARTE MAISON   tart prepared in the manner of the
    restaurant
TARTE MÉGIN   cream cheese tart

TARTE MOUGIN   tart with eggs, cream and cream cheese
TARTE TATIN   caramelized upside down apple pie, served warm
TARTELETTES   little tarts filled with various ingredients
TARTINE   slice of bread
TARTOUFFE   potato
TARTOUILLAT   apple tart
TASSE   cup
TASTE-VIN   wine tasting cup
TEMPLE GLACÉ À LA MARTINIQUAISE   mold of ice cream with rum and chocolate
TENDRONS DE VEAU   braised veal
TERRINE   earthenware container for baking meat, game, fish or vegetable mixture
TERRINE AUX AROMATES   herb pâté
TERRINE D'ANGUILLE   eel cooked in an earthenware container
TERRINE D'OIE   finely ground goosemeat, usually served as an appetizer
TERRINE DE BOEUF   beef stew with vegetables and wine
TERRINE DE BROCHET   finely ground pike, usually served as an appetizer
TERRINE DE CAILLE   quail cooked in an earthenware container
TERRINE DE CANARD   duck cooked in an earthenware container
TERRINE DE FAISAN   pheasant cooked in an earthenware container
TERRINE DE FOIE   liver cooked in an earthenware container
TERRINE DE FOIES DE VOLAILLE   chicken liver in an earthenware container
TERRINE DE GIBIER   wild game pâté
TERRINE DE GRIVES   thrush cooked in an earthenware container
TERRINE DE JAMBON   finely ground ham, combined with cream and sherry

TERRINE DE LAPIN   rabbit pâté

TERRINE DE MOUTON   finely ground mutton combined with spices and cream

TERRINE DE PERDREAU   partridge cooked in an earthenware container

TERRINE DE PORC   pork pâté with ham

TERRINE DE VEAU   veal pâté with ham

TERRINE DE VOLAILLE   chicken cooked in an earthenware container

TERRINE MAISON   mixture of chicken, goose livers or pork

TÊTE DE VEAU   calf's head

TÊTE DE VEAU À LA VINAIGRETTE   calf's head served in oil and vinegar

TÉTRAS   grouse

THÉ   tea

THÉ AU CITRON   tea with lemon

THÉ AU LAIT   tea with milk

THÉ NATURE   plain tea

THON   tuna

THOURIN POTAGE   milk-onion soup with cheese on bread

THYM   thyme, aromatic herb

TIAN   vegetable mixture cooked in an earthenware dish

TIÈDE   lukewarm

TIMBALE   round baking mold or mixture prepared in such a mold, often with pastry cover

TIMBALE D'ÉPINARDS   molded spinach custard

TIMBALE DE FOIES DE VOLAILLE   chicken liver mold

TIMBALE DE FRUITS   pastry with apricot jam and cooked fruits on top

TIMBALE DE JAMBON   molded ham custard

TIORO   fish stew with tomato, onion and garlic

TIRE-BOUCHON   corkscrew

TIREZ   pull

TISANE   herb tea

TOILETTES   toilets

TOMATE   tomato
TOMATE À L'ANTIBOISE   marinated tomato stuffed with tuna
TOMATE AU THON À LA MAYONNAISE   tomato stuffed with tuna and mayonnaise
TOMATE FARCIE   stuffed tomato
TOMATE GRILLÉE   grilled tomato
TOMATE POLONAISE   breaded baked tomatoes
TOMATE PROVENÇALE   tomato with breadcrumbs and garlic
TOMME   mild soft cheese
TOMME ARLÉSIENNE   soft, sheep's milk cheese, very creamy
TOMME AU MARC DE RAISIN   semi-hard cheese
TOMME DE SAVOIE   very mild, semi-soft cheese
TOPINAMBOUR   Jerusalem artichoke
TORTUE   turtle, tortoise
TORTUE VÉRITABLE, SOUPE DE   real turtle soup
TÔT-FAIT   spongecake with lemon
TOTELOTS   hot noodle salad
TOULIA   onion soup with tomatoes, leeks, cheese and garlic
TOURANGELLE, À LA   fried croutons topped with eggs poached in red wine
TOURNEDOS   center of beef filet, grilled or sautéed
TOURNEDOS À LA BÉARNAISE   grilled steak served on toast with béarnaise sauce
TOURNEDOS À LA PÉRIGOURDINE   cuts of steak with truffles
TOURNEDOS ALEXANDRA   steak sautéed with artichoke hearts
TOURNEDOS ARLÉSIEN   steak sautéed, served with fried eggplant and tomatoes
TOURNEDOS AUX CHAMPIGNONS   beef fillets with mushrooms
TOURNEDOS CHASSEUR   pan-fried steak in wine, mushrooms and tomato paste

TOURNEDOS CLAMART   pan-fried seeak with fresh peas

TOURNEDOS DES GOURMETS   steak fried in sherry, served with goose liver

TOURNEDOS GRILLÉ   grilled tournedos

TOURNEDOS MAÎTRE D'HÔTEL   grilled or pan-fried

TOURNEDOS ROSSINI   sautéed tournedos garnished with liver and truffles

TOURON   candy of almonds, pistachio and crystallized fruit

TOURTE   pastry shell filled with foods and then sliced

TOURTE DE CANETON   duck baked in a pie

TOURTE DE MOUTON   mutton pie

TOURTE LORRAINE   tart with pork and veal in cream

TOURTEAU AU FROMAGE   goat's milk cheesecake

TOURTELETTE   individual filled pastry

TOURTIÈRE   chicken pie

TOUT COMPRIS   all-inclusive price

TRANCHE   slice

TRANCHE DE CABILLAUD   codfish steaks

TRANCHE DE JAMBON ROSE-MARIE   ham slices in cream sauce

TRANCHE NAPOLITAINE   ice cream and crystallized fruit

TRIPE   stomach lining of a cow

TRIPE À LA MODE DE CAEN   beef tripe, onions, leeks, cooked in cider and Calvados brandy

TRIPE FERTE MACE   tripe cooked on skewers

TRIPLE SEC   orange liqueur

TRIPOTCHA   spicy pudding

TRIPOUX   mutton tripe

TROUFFE   slang for potato

TRUFFADE   fried potato mashed with cheese, tomatoes, bacon and garlic

TRUFFE   truffle, in the onion family, used for flavoring

TRUFFE EN CROÛTE   truffle and goose liver in pastry

TRUFFIAT   potato cake

TRUITE   trout

TRUITE AMANDINE   trout served with slivers of toasted almonds
TRUITE ARC-EN CIEL   rainbow trout
TRUITE AU BLEU   trout poached in vinegar bouillion
TRUITE DE LAC   lake trout
TRUITE DE RIVIÈRE   river trout
TRUITE GOURMET   trout with mayonnaise and artichokes
TRUITE MONTBARDOISE   trout stuffed with spinach
TRUITE MONTGOLFIER   boneless trout, white wine and lobster sauce
TRUITE SAUMONÉE   salmon trout
TRUITE SAUMONÉE EN GELÉE   cold salmon trout in aspic
TRUITE VIVANTE   trout alive till immediately before cooking
TRUITES AUX AMANDES   trout with almonds
TUILE   delicate almond flavored cookie
TURBOT   flat sea fish like flounder
TURBOT AU CHAMPAGNE   poached in white wine or champagne
TURBOTIN   turbot
TVA   tax added to bill

V

V.S.O.P. VERY SPECIAL OLD PALE   cognac aged 5 years
VACHERIN   meringue case for dessert creams, ice creams or fruit and berry mixtures
VACHERIN ABONDANCE   runny, mild cheese
VACHERIN DU MONT D'OR   firm, mild flavored cows' milk cheese
VACHERIN GLACÉ   ice cream dessert with meringue
VALENÇAY   strong creamy goat cheese
VALENCE, ORANGE DE   Valencia orange
VALENCIENNE   tomato, rice, mushrooms, tongue and cheese

VALLÉE D'AUGE   garnish of cooked apples and cream
VANGEREN   type of carp
VANILLE   vanilla
VAPEUR   steamed
VARENNE   herb mayonnaise
VARIÉ   assorted or varied
VAUCLUSIENNE   fried in olive oil, served with lemon juice
VAUDOISE   variety of carp
VEAU   veal
VEAU À LA FLAMANDE   veal braised with fruits
VEAU, BLANQUETTE DE   veal stew
VEAU CUSTINE   fried veal chops with tomato sauce
VEAU, FRICADELLES DE   ground veal patties
VEAU HOLSTEIN   sautéed veal with fried eggs and anchovies
VEAU, JARRET DE   veal shank
VEAU, POITRINE DE   stuffed breast of veal
VEAU, RIS DE   veal sweetbreads
VEAU RÔTI   roast veal
VEAU, SAUTÉ DE   veal stew
VEAU SYLVIE   veal roasted with ham and cheese
VEAU, TENDRON DE   breast of veal stewed with vegetables
VÉGÉTARIENNE, CUISINE   vegetarian cooking
VELOUTÉ   a sauce, soup or dish having a smooth, creamy taste, also see Crème
VELOUTÉ D'OIGNON   cream of onion soup
VELOUTÉ DE TOMATE   cream of tomato soup
VELOUTÉ DE VOLAILLE   cream of chicken soup
VELOUTÉ DE VOLAILLE LA SÉNÉGALAISE   curried turkey soup, hot or cold
VENAISON   venison
VÉNUS   sea cockle, a shellfish
VERMICELLE   very thin spaghetti
VERRE   glass
VERVEINE   herb tea

VIANDE   meat
VIANDE CHAUDE   hot meat
VIANDE FROIDE   cold meat
VIANDE SÉCHÉE   cured dried beef
VICHY   a brand of mineral water
VICHYSSOISE   chilled, pureed, leek and potato soup
VICHYSSOISE À LA RUSSE   cold leek and potato soup
   with beets and sour cream
VIEUX PUANT   soft, very spicy cheese
VIGNOBLE   vineyard
VIN   wine
VIN BLANC   white wine
VIN CHAMBRÉ   wine at room temperature
VIN CONSOMMATION COURANTE   plain table wine
VIN DE TABLE   plain table wine
VIN DOUX   dessert wine
VIN DOUX NATUREL   sweet wine
VIN DU PAYS   local wine
VIN GRIS   pale red-pink wine
VIN LIMITE QUALITÉ SUPÉRIEURE VDQS   second
   category wine
VIN MAISON   house wine
VIN MOUSSEUX   sparkling wine
VIN, ORANGE AU   orange sections in white wine
VIN ORDINAIRE   everyday table wine
VIN ROSÉ   pink wine
VIN ROUGE   red wine
VIN SEC   dry wine
VINAIGRE   vinegar
VINAIGRETTE   French dressing for green salads,
   combination salads, and marinades
VOL-AU-VENT   large puff pastry shell
VOLAILLE   poultry, also see poulet
VOLAILLE FROIDE   cold poultry
VOTRE SANTÉ, À   "to your health", a drinking toast
VRILLES DE LA VIGNE   vine cuttings, usually prepared
   with olive oil

W

WATERZOOI   chicken or fish stew in creamy sauce
WILLIAM   sweet pear

X

XAVIER   creamy rice soup
XÉRÈS   sherry

Y

YAOURT   yogurt
YAOURT À LA CONFITURE   with preserves

Z

ZESTE   peel of orange or lemon
ZEWELMAI   onion and cream flan
ZIMINU   fish soup
ZINGARA   with tomato, ham and mushrooms
ZUCCHINI   Italian squash